ORTHOPEDIC JOINT MOBILIZATION AND MANIPULATION

AN EVIDENCE-BASED APPROACH

Robert C. Manske, PT, DPT, MEd, SCS, ATC, CSCS
Wichita State University

B.J. Lehecka, DPT
Wichita State University

Michael P. Reiman, PT, DPT, MEd, OCS, SCS, ATC, FAAOMPT, CSCS
Duke University Medical Center

Janice K. Loudon, PT, PhD, SCS, ATC, CSCS
Rockhurst University

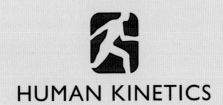

HUMAN KINETICS

Library of Congress Cataloging-in-Publication Data

Names: Manske, Robert C., author. | Lehecka, B. J., 1982- author. | Reiman, Michael P., 1965- author. | Loudon, Janice K. (Janice Kaye), 1959- author.
Title: Orthopedic joint mobilization and manipulation : an evidence-based approach / Robert C. Manske, B.J. Lehecka, Michael P. Reiman, Janice K. Loudon.
Description: Champaign, IL : Human Kinetics, [2019] | Includes bibliographical references and index.
Identifiers: LCCN 2017023781 (print) | LCCN 2017023190 (ebook) | ISBN 9781492544968 (e-book) | ISBN 9781492544951 (print)
Subjects: | MESH: Manipulation, Orthopedic--methods | Joints--physiology | Manipulation, Spinal--methods | Range of Motion, Articular--physiology | Evidence-Based Medicine
Classification: LCC RD731 (print) | LCC RD731 (ebook) | NLM WB 535 | DDC 617.4/7--dc23
LC record available at https://lccn.loc.gov/2017023781

ISBN: 978-1-4925-4495-1 (print)

The web addresses cited in this text were current as of May 2018, unless otherwise noted.

Senior Acquisitions Editor: Joshua J. Stone; **Developmental and Managing Editor:** Amanda S. Ewing; **Copyeditor:** John Wentworth; **Indexer:** Nancy Ball; **Permissions Manager:** Dalene Reeder; **Senior Graphic Designers:** Keri Evans and Joe Buck; **Cover Designer:** Keri Evans; **Cover Design Associate:** Susan Rothermel Allen; **Photographs (cover):** © Human Kinetics; **Photographs (interior):** © Human Kinetics; **Photographer:** Jason Allen; **Visual Production Assistant:** Joyce Brumfield; **Photo Production Manager:** Jason Allen; **Senior Art Manager:** Kelly Hendren; **Illustrations:** © Human Kinetics; **Printer:** Walsworth

The video contents of this product are licensed for educational public performance for viewing by a traditional (live) audience, via closed circuit television, or via computerized local area networks within a single building or geographically unified campus. To request a license to broadcast these contents to a wider audience—for example, throughout a school district or state, or on a television station—please contact your sales representative **(www.HumanKinetics.com/SalesRepresentatives)**.

Printed in the United States of America

10 9 8 7 6 5 4 3 2 1

The paper in this book was manufactured using responsible forestry methods.

Human Kinetics

P.O. Box 5076
Champaign, IL 61825-5076
Website: www.HumanKinetics.com

In the United States, email info@hkusa.com or call 800-747-4457.
In Canada, email info@hkcanada.com.
In the United Kingdom/Europe, email hk@hkeurope.com.

For information about Human Kinetics' coverage in other areas of the world, please visit our website: **www.HumanKinetics.com**

E6967

CONTENTS

PART I   Introduction

PART II   Mobilization and Manipulation of the Craniomandibular Complex and Spine

TREATMENT FINDER

Temporomandibular Joint

Cervical Spine

Thoracic Spine

Lumbar Spine and Pelvis

Shoulder Joint

Elbow Joint

Wrist and Hand

Hip Joint

Knee Joint

Ankle Joint

Foot

Self-Mobilizations

PREFACE

The purpose of this book is to provide educators, clinicians, and students of pre-professional physical therapy and osteopathic medical programs a comprehensive evidence-based text on the clinical application of joint thrust and nonthrust procedures. This book is designed for physical therapists, osteopathic doctors, educators, and students of pre-professional therapy and osteopathic programs charged with treatment of patients with musculoskeletal joint pain and dysfunction. The language and content of the text is easy to follow for use in the classroom, lab, clinical, or professional workshop setting. The text provides the reader an appreciation for the current evidence and theory supporting the clinical application of joint thrust/nonthrust for clients experiencing symptoms across a wide range of musculoskeletal ailments related to pain, limited joint mobility, and dysfunction. Joint manipulation and mobilization has been practiced for more than 40 years. This form of joint manipulation and mobilization is a popular form of manipulation used by a large percentage of physical therapy programs in the United States. It is one of the easiest techniques to understand and apply in clinical practice. This book offers the reader a straightforward approach based on traditional anatomical structure and function as well as current evidence.

The text provides a comprehensive overview of the literature supporting the use of joint mobilization and manipulation and manual therapy as well as complementary explanations of the literature, concepts, and theories to bolster the reader's understanding of how thrust and nonthrust techniques work to eliminate pain and re-establish normal joint motion and function. Readers are instructed on how to determine arthrokinematic joint dysfunction to be treated with joint mobilization/manipulation. Additionally, the text provides the aspiring manual therapist with easy-to-apply methods for treatment of common musculoskeletal conditions.

Unique to this book is anatomical artwork overlaid on pictures of the clinical techniques. This is designed to give readers improved visualization of the techniques' intentions and to guide hand placement and procedures. Relevant clinical tips exist in each chapter to further readers' understanding of techniques.

Part I introduces the basic science behind joint mobilization and manipulation, including indications, general joint kinesiology, and other information. Part II describes specific thrust and nonthrust techniques for the entire spine and temporomandibular joint. Part III details techniques for the upper extremity. Part IV describes techniques for the lower extremity. Finally, the appendix presents 26 self-mobilizations. We hope the clear, organized, and well-illustrated descriptions of these techniques will benefit all readers as well as the clients they treat.

Student Resources

Students will benefit significantly by completing the 11 case studies, with questions showing treatments for patients suffering from various musculoskeletal conditions, in the accompanying web study guide. In addition to the case studies, there are 60 videos of treatment techniques. The web study guide is available at www.HumanKinetics.com/OrthopedicJoint MobilizationAndManipulation.

Instructor Resources

Two ancillaries are available to instructors:

- Instructor guide: This guide details how to best use the various ancillaries and includes a sample syllabus and ideas for lab activities and class projects.
- Chapter quizzes: Each chapter is supported by a ready-made chapter quiz to assess student understanding of the main concepts of the chapter.

These ancillaries are available at www.Human Kinetics.com/OrthopedicJointMobilizationAnd Manipulation.

ACKNOWLEDGMENTS

This book started out as handouts used by several of the authors in their respective physical therapy programs. It has become a much more valuable and fine-tuned resource thanks to the expert help and guidance of Josh Stone and Amanda Ewing at Human Kinetics. Without their editorial assistance and persistent pushing to stay on time, it would never be the book it is at present. We would also like to acknowledge Heidi Richter for her excellent work with the medical overlays for the photos in our textbook. The overlays are a crucial part of this textbook because they allow the reader to better understand hand placement for mobilization and manipulation.

We would like to thank all our mentors, prior students, and administrations at our respective universities who have helped us develop the skill set needed to formulate a textbook of this nature.

Last, but not least, we would like to thank our families and friends for allowing us the time away from them needed to write this textbook.

Introduction

Part I of this text includes chapter 1, which covers the basic science behind joint mobilization/manipulation, and chapter 2, which presents general application guidelines. Chapter 1 details principles of joint mobilization and manipulation techniques that are commonly held within the field, including clinicians who apply joint mobilization and manipulation on their clients. These foundational principles are key for the reader to comprehend when implementing the techniques outlined in subsequent chapters. Chapter 1 concludes with various proposed mechanisms for joint mobilization and manipulation.

Chapter 2 provides general guidelines regarding the application of joint mobilization/manipulation. These guidelines primarily include detail on joint play (arthrokinematic) assessment, assessment of joint end-feel, and description of capsular versus noncapsular patterns. Joint mobilization parameters, variables, and duration of applications are also covered in this chapter. Finally, this chapter describes precautions, indications, and contraindications for the reader.

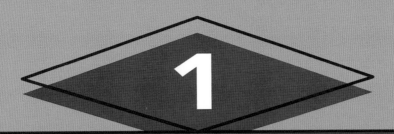

1

BASIC SCIENCE BEHIND JOINT MOBILIZATION AND MANIPULATION

LEARNING OBJECTIVES

After completing this chapter, you will be able to do the following:

- Define the basic concepts surrounding joint mobilization and manipulation
- Describe the principles of joint mobilization and manipulation
- Explain convex and concave rules
- Describe osteokinematic and arthrokinematic movements
- Understand which effect you want to use mobilization and manipulation for when treating a musculoskeletal condition

In order to provide appropriate care to clients, clinicians must understand the rudimentary concepts and principles underlying joint mobilization and manipulation. This chapter presents basic information that all clinicians require to be able to determine and apply appropriate treatment for clients with limited joint mobility caused by restricted capsular structures. The chapter thus serves as an introduction to the primary purpose of this text—to present and describe mobilization techniques that are used to restore joints' passive accessory motion.

A healthy joint is one that will move without inherent immobility. Movements at synovial joint surfaces provide a stimulus to produce synovial fluid and nourish articular structures such as disc, meniscus, and cartilage. Normal movement at a joint allows gliding of capsular structures that helps to retain their form and structure. Numerous negative physiological consequences occur through immobilization or loss of movement. These include fatty infiltration, articular adhesions, and physiologic changes to tissues such as capsules, ligaments, and tendons.

History and Legislation

The origins of manual therapy likely predate recorded history. Humans have sought musculoskeletal treatments that involve traction, joint mobilization, joint manipulation, or a combination of these. Traditionally, physical therapists have included traction and mobilization procedures as part of their routine clinical practice. As basic medical sciences and knowledge about the musculoskeletal system has advanced, so has our knowledge in how to treat these ailments.

Legislation regarding support for the use of mobilization and, especially, manipulation is transforming. Legislation currently differs from one state to the next, requiring physical therapists to remain updated regarding their state's directives regarding mobilization and manipulation to ensure they are practicing in consistency with regulations. In several states, legislation is currently being challenged.

Mobilization and Manipulation

Joint mobilization, also known as nonthrust manipulation, is the treatment of motion restriction of accessory joint play. This is a treatment of passive movements at the joint interface. According to the *Guide to Physical Therapist Practice*, manipulation and mobilization can be used interchangeably and are defined as "a continuum of skilled passive movements to joints and/or related soft tissues that are applied at varying speeds and amplitudes, including a small amplitude/high velocity therapeutic movement" (APTA, 2017). Physical therapists routinely use manual, passive manipulation and mobilization to treat accessory joint motion limitations, correct dysfunctional movement patterns, restore joint motion or mobility, and/or decrease pain associated with joint structures (Barak, Rosen, and Sofer, 1990). These passive treatments are generally well tolerated and not uncomfortable for the client. The vast majority of the treatment techniques presented in this text are *local* joint mobilizations specific to a particular segment or region of a joint—as opposed to *regional* joint mobilizations, which are applied to more than 1 area, segment, or component (Maher and Latimer, 1993).

The International Federation of Orthopaedic Manipulative Physical Therapists (IFOMPT) provides the following definitions:

- *Manipulation*: A passive, high-velocity, low-amplitude thrust applied to a joint complex within its anatomical limit with the intent to restore optimal motion, function, and/or to reduce pain.
- *Mobilization*: A manual therapy technique comprising a continuum of skilled passive movements to the joint complex applied at varying speeds and amplitudes; these may include a small-amplitude/high-velocity therapeutic movement (manipulation) with the intent to restore optimal motion, function, and/or to reduce pain.

Slightly complicating matters, others in the field use the term *thrust manipulation* in reference to IFOMPT's concept of manipulation, and *nonthrust manipulation* as synonymous with IFOMPT's concept of mobilization (Rushton et al., 2016).

Before proceeding further, a few basics should be fully absorbed. Mobilization is often performed to increase range of motion. Range of motion involves physiologic active or passive movements performed normally through 1 of the cardinal planes of motion. The cardinal planes of motion are flexion and extension, abduction and adduction, and internal and external rotation. An *osteokinematic* movement of a joint can be seen by anyone. When someone raises her shoulder, for example, even a nontrained person can see the elevation. An osteokinematic motion is also sometimes referred to as a classical motion, a physiologic motion, or a traditional movement. With training, these motions can even be measured accurately with a goniometer. Osteokinematic motions can occur either actively, through volitional control, or passively by someone else. A much more complex movement is the *arthrokinematic* motion, which is the actual movement isolated at the joint level at the bone ends. These motions occur without regard to the larger osteokinematic motion of the joint. Arthrokinematic movements are known as accessory movements and are not under volitional control. These movements are specific to the paired articular joint surfaces (Barak, Rosen, and Sofer, 1990; Wooden, 1989). Osteokinematic and arthrokinematic movements are discussed further in the Joint Movements section.

Joint Congruency and Position

Joint congruency involves the amount of surface contact between 2 opposing joint surfaces. A joint that is congruent has both surfaces in close approximation with a relatively large amount of contact between the 2 ends of the joints (MacConaill and Basmajian, 1969). In synovial joints, the ends of the 2 bone surfaces are usually covered with hyaline articular cartilage. If the joint surface is more convex in nature there is usually more articular cartilage at the center, whereas on a concave articular surface more cartilage is found near the periphery. When both surfaces appear flat, the larger surface should be considered to be convex (Barak, Rosen, and Sofer, 1990). A joint has greater congruency when in the closed packed position than when in the loose packed or resting positions. A joint is in the closed packed position when the articular surfaces are aligned, the joint capsular structures and surrounding ligaments are taut, and there is minimal joint volume remaining. This is the position in which the joint is most stable and is commonly used for testing ligament and capsular integrity. However, because there is minimal to no joint play in this position, it is not used for joint mobilizations. Because the close packed position is one of stability, joint mobilizations would not need to be performed here. An example of a closed packed position is full extension at the knee or the elbow. In this position, these joints are extremely stable, with little passive movement available at the joint surface.

The phalanges of the fingers are in the closed packed position when the fingers are fully extended. In this position, the capsule and collateral ligaments are taut, allowing little to no joint passive movement. Performance of joint mobilization in this position would be useless, as no further motion into extension can occur once the closed packed position has been attained.

Any position other than closed packed is a loose packed position. The resting position is the position, within loose packed positions, in which the joint capsule and ligaments are most relaxed and loose. This position allows the maximum amount of joint play and is thus the best position for testing passive mobility. Using the phalanges again as a reference, the loose packed position is when the joint is in slight flexion. This is also the position in which a painful, stiff, and dysfunctional joint may move the easiest. However, a joint would have to be extremely limited, almost ankylosed, to be limited to movement only at the resting position.

Joint Movements

A joint with unrestricted movement can move freely within its range of motion. As described earlier, osteokinematic movements are those that are under one's volition and easily detected by the naked eye. By contrast, arthrokinematic movements occur at the joint level and are not easily seen by the naked eye. Arthrokinematic movements involve the movement of 2 joint surfaces and are not under voluntary control. These "accessory" motions—called rolls, glides, and spins—are prerequisite for full, unrestricted motion. A roll occurs similar to a tire on pavement. During rolling of a joint, a new portion of the joint comes in contact with the opposite joint surface as the joint moves through its range of motion. A glide is similar to a tire sliding on ice when the brakes are hit. Here, 1 part of a moving joint is in contact with multiple points on the opposing surface. A spin is when the joint surface spins or rotates along a joint surface, such as when a child spins a top.

Convex and Concave Rules

Most human synovial articular joint surfaces are either convex or concave, although in a few cases the joint surfaces are not exactly either shape (Wooden, 1989). An example of a convex structure is the large humeral head, while a concave structure is the glenoid fossa. In some cases, it is not always easy to determine which portion of a joint is convex and which is concave. In these cases, where the shape of the joint surface is not convex or concave, there is usually a disc or structure within the joint to provide and modify the contour to make it more cohesive.

Convex and concave rules are used to describe the arthrokinematic movement that occurs in a normal moving joint without restrictions (figure 1.1). One rule states: "When the concave surface is stationary and the convex surface is moving, the gliding movement in the joint occurs in the direction opposite the bone movement" (Barak, Rosen, and Sofer, 1990, p. 202). Conversely, the second rule states: "When the convex surface is fixed while the concave surface is moving, the gliding motion occurs in the same direction as the bone movement" (Ibid.). It is worthy of mention, however, that some findings suggest limitations in the clinical utility of this second rule. Numerous studies indicate that the glenohumeral joint does not always move as a ball-and-socket joint, but occasionally displays only translatory movements during pathology (Baeyens, Van Roy, De Schepper, Declercq, and Clarijs, 2001; McClure and Flowers, 1992), so mobilizations according to this rule may be worthy of scrutiny (Johnson, Godges, Zimmerman, and Ounanian, 2007). Reasonable data support that this process is predictive in the knee and ankle as well (Frankel, Burstein, and Brooks, 1971; Sammarco, Burstein, and Frankel, 1973).

Effects of Mobilization and Manipulation

Clinicians use joint mobilization and manipulation for 2 main indications: joint pain and joint hypomobility. Three main categories of effects of mobilization or manipulation are described here: mechanical, neurophysiological, and psychological.

Mechanical Effects

The mechanical effects of joint mobilization relate to the restoration of normal joint mobility or range of motion. This includes flexibility and mobility of capsular and other soft tissue structures such as ligaments and tendons. Following injury and immobilization, soft tissues can become shortened and limit overall joint mobility. Adequate force must be applied to the tissues to create mechanical effects. Higher grade mobilizations may increase the joint mobility back to normal by restoring relative amounts of play in the once-restricted joint motion. Another theory of mechanical effect is the releasing or freeing of the facet joint meniscoid entrapment. A meniscoid entrapment may include a locking caused by entrapment of a facet joint meniscoid in a groove formed in the articular cartilage or by a meniscus piece that has broken free and formed a loose body that is entrapped (Lewitt, 1985). These meniscoids can become extremely painful sources of dysfunction. Fortunately, either gapping or an isometric movement that pulls the facet laterally can theoretically dislodge the impingement; the result can be immediate pain relief and improvement of joint motion. Current evidence supports only transient biomechanical effects on studies quantifying motion (Colloca, Keller, Harrison, Moore, Gunzburg, and Harrison, 2006; Coppieters and Alshami, 2007; Coppieters and Butler, 2007; Gal, Herzog, Kawchuk, Conway, and Zhang, 1997) but not a lasting positional change (Hsieh, Vicenzino, Yang, Hu, and Yang, 2002; Tullberg, Blomberg, Branth, and Johnsson, 1998). Neurophysiological and psychological effects should therefore be strongly considered.

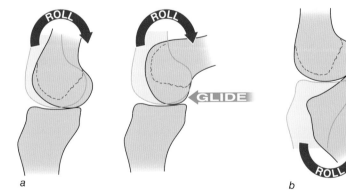

Figure 1.1 *(a)* Convex-on-concave arthrokinematics. *(b)* Concave-on-convex arthrokinematics.

Neurophysiological Effects

Applications of joint mobilizations and manipulation have been reported to create both local and distal neurophysiological effects (Bialosky, Bishop, and Bialosky, 2009; Bishop, Beneciuk, and George, 2011; Coranoda, Gay, and Bialosky, 2012; George, Bishop, and Bialosky, 2006). These effects may be especially enhanced when using the spine as the region of mobilization or manipulation application. Spinal soft tissues are highly innervated and may provide a large degree of afferent input into the central nervous system (Groen, Baljet, and Drukker, 1990). This input can come from multiple sources such as type I and II mechanoreceptors and free nerve endings found in cervical spine facet joints and muscle spindles of the cervical spine. Similar mechanisms might be seen in the remainder of the spine, but the number of nerve endings may be lower and less consistent in lower levels of the spine (McLain and Pickar, 1998). Movement such as mobilization or manipulation will fire these receptors and provide input to the central nervous system. These nerve receptors terminate in the spinal cord synapsing in the ventral and dorsal horn to signal proprioceptive and nociceptive information (Bolton, 1998).

Animal and human models have shown that the periaqueductal gray area of the midbrain is key for control of mediation of endogenous analgesia (Cannon, Prieto, and Lee, 1982; Hosobuchi, Adams, and Linchitz 1977; Reynolds, 1969). The periaqueductal gray area is in coordination with a complex network of systems including the nociceptive system, the autonomic nervous system, and the motor system. It has also been shown that type I and II mechanoreceptors from joints, muscles, and tendons project to the periaqueductal gray area (Yezierski, 1991). Evidence via postmanipulation sympathetic response combined with analgesia in symptomatic and asymptomatic subjects suggests a neurophysiologic response to spinal manipulation via mechanoreceptors (Wright, 1995). These effects may lie in the stimulation of the descending pain-inhibitory system of the central nervous system from midbrain to spinal cord.

Controversy persists regarding whether analgesic effects from mobilization and manipulation occur following treatment. Some reports suggest that mobilization or manipulation may stimulate a release of endogenous opioid peptides that bind to nervous system receptor sites, producing analgesia. Vernon and colleagues found increased levels of plasma beta-endorphin following manipulation, but these levels diminished to normal levels after only 15 minutes (Vernon, Dhami, Howley, et al., 1986). Controversy continues, as others have not succeeded in documenting these increased levels of endorphin compared to control groups (Christian, Stanton, and Sissons, 1998; Sanders, Reinnert, and Tepe, 1990).

The neurophysiological effect may also include a change in muscle activation patterns in which the motor system may be inhibited. The ability of mobilization and manipulation to inhibit muscle may vary depending on technique, location and nature of pain, and even the given muscles targeted with the manipulation. If mobilization or manipulation affects muscles, the neurophysiologic effects most likely occur locally at the targeted joint or region and the corresponding innervation distally associated with the shared innervation. The effects desired from performing the mobilization or manipulation are to increase facilitation of the deeper, more local muscles that assist with neuromuscular control of the area and, ideally, to inhibit the more superficial, global muscles that may be causing pain due to increased guarding of the joint or segments involved.

Psychological Effects

At least in the spinal model, evidence of improvement of psychological outcomes following manipulation is limited. In a meta-analysis, Williams, Hendry, Lewis, and colleagues (2007) reviewed 129 randomized controlled trials of spinal manipulation and identified 12 studies reporting psychological outcomes. These studies suggest that spinal manipulation may improve psychological outcomes compared to verbal interventions. Further, other variables, such as clinician and client expectations, may also play a role in the degree to which symptoms improve (Cross, Leach, Fawkes, and Moore, 2015; Riley, Bialosky, Cote, Swanson, Tafuto, Sizer, and Brismée, 2015). The greatest effect seems to be in those with a positive attitude and an expectation that the intervention will be helpful.

Evidence for Joint Mobilization

Chapters 3 through 13 conclude with a table listing available evidence for the use of mobilization or manipulation techniques for the region discussed in that chapter. Readers will thus be able to clearly deduce the level of study, the quality, including number of subjects or studies reviewed, outcomes measured, and a brief synopsis of the results. These tables are provided to help bridge the gap between clinical practice and best available evidence of benefit or usefulness. For some regions, high-quality studies demonstrate usefulness of manual therapy. For other regions, evidence to support the use of manual therapy is scant, or nonexistent.

Summary

Understanding the basic concepts of joint mobilization and manipulation is essential to appreciate the importance of these techniques. The various methods of mobilization and manipulation allow clinicians to use the one they feel would be optimal in the treatment of a musculoskeletal condition. Understanding the different types of joint movements—both voluntary (osteokinematic) and involuntary accessory (arthrokinematic) movements—is critical to properly applying the many techniques described in subsequent chapters. Joint mobilization and manipulation will create multiple types of effects for those on whom these techniques are applied. Our understanding of these effects will evolve as research on mobilization and manipulation techniques continues.

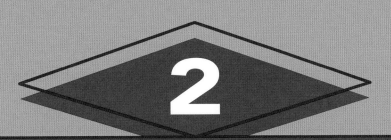

GENERAL APPLICATION GUIDELINES

CHAPTER OBJECTIVES

After completing this chapter, you will be able to do the following:

- Explain general examination procedures and how joint end-feels and capsular patterns relate to manual therapy
- Describe parameters for the clinical application of joint thrusts and nonthrusts, including dosage and other variables
- Identify indications, contraindications, and other safety considerations for thrust and nonthrust techniques

Several basics about joint motion, joint capsules, thrust and nonthrust parameters, and indications/contraindications for thrusts and nonthrusts must be understood before applying the techniques in chapters 3 through 13. Clinicians should have a strong understanding of end-feels, including normal and abnormal end-feels. They should be aware of the target joint's capsular pattern to aid their choice of thrust and nonthrust techniques. Also, for client safety, clinicians must screen for precautions and contraindications to the techniques described in this book.

General Examination

Joint thrusts and nonthrusts should be performed only following thorough subjective and objective examinations. These preliminary examinations serve to guide clinicians to the most appropriate thrust and nonthrust techniques for their clients. The subjective examination should precede the objective examination and provide the clinician with a short list of potential client diagnoses. During the subjective examination, clinicians should determine whether the client has previously received thrust or nonthrust techniques for their impairment. If so, details about which techniques were used, by whom, and with what outcomes will help guide subsequent treatment. For optimal outcomes, clients should feel comfortable with their clinician and the prescribed treatments. The subjective examination is an ideal point to begin building rapport with clients and deciphering which techniques will be most appropriate.

The objective examination serves to confirm findings of the subjective examination and further narrow the list of potential client diagnoses. It often includes goniometric measurements, manual muscle testing or other muscle-testing procedures, special testing, and palpation. Goniometry during active and passive range of motion allows clinicians to distinguish between muscular limitations and limitations caused by capsule tightening or other anatomical restrictions. Muscle testing, while not directly related to thrust or nonthrust techniques, informs clinicians of painful, irritated, or otherwise damaged muscular tissue. Similar to information gathered during palpation, information received during muscle testing may direct clinicians' hand placements and client positioning during the techniques described in this text. Select special tests are intended to determine specifically whether arthrokinematic motion is limited and thrust or nonthrust techniques are indicated. Finally, if a joint's arthrokinematics are not assessed during special testing or goniometry, the palpation section of the objective examination should be used to learn the arthrokinematics of the target and surrounding areas of a client's impairment. Clinicians can determine whether thrust or nonthrust techniques are indicated only after the aforementioned procedures are performed.

End-Feels

Dr. James Cyriax, DO, originally coined the concept of *end-feel* to describe the resistance felt at the limit of a joint's range of motion by a clinician (Cyriax, 1975). Multiple types of end-feels have been described, including normal end-feels (bony, soft tissue approximation, and tissue stretch) and abnormal end-feels (muscle spasm, capsular, springy block, and empty) (Reiman, 2016). Bony and soft tissue approximation end-feels, such as normal elbow extension and elbow flexion, respectively, are not the target of thrust and nonthrust techniques.

A tissue stretch end-feel is similar to the abnormal capsular end-feel, except the capsular end-feel is a firm stop in an unexpected location. The capsular end-feel is typically thicker than the tissue stretch end-feel, and it typically accompanies a decrease in normal joint range of motion. Capsular end-feels are the targets of both thrust and nonthrust techniques. It is assumed that if a limitation is caused by capsular tightness, thrusts

and nonthrusts will aid normalization of the joint's end-feel and range of motion.

A muscle spasm end-feel (e.g., spasticity) or empty end-feel (limitation of motion due to pain) prohibit thrust and nonthrust techniques from clinicians, or at least strongly limit their effectiveness. Modalities and other relaxation or pain-relieving maneuvers may help clinicians decrease muscle spasm or empty end-feels for further evaluation of joint end-feels and possible prescription of thrust or nonthrust techniques.

Capsular Patterns

Dr. Cyriax also developed the concept of capsular patterns (Cyriax, 1975). The capsule constructed of fibrous connective tissue helps to maintain the integrity of a synovial joint. Injury directly affecting the capsule can result in pain and loss of passive range of motion (PROM) in a recognizable pattern referred to as a capsular pattern. Each diarthrodial joint has a characteristic and reproducible capsular pattern as defined by Dr. Cyriax. An example of a capsular pattern for the glenohumeral joint is loss of external rotation to a greater extent followed by loss of abduction and slight loss of internal rotation.

Knowledge of the capsular pattern can improve diagnostic abilities by identifying the tissue that is restricting motion. The pattern could be a result of a shortened capsule that may occur in arthrosis or any type of arthritis that affects the capsule and synovium. Acute conditions affecting only the synovium cause a capsular limitation of motion because of the muscular spasm protecting the capsule. Periods of prolonged immobilization may result in a shortened capsule and a capsular restriction of motion.

Capsular patterns are based on theory, and in certain joints the capsular patterns may be different or inconsistent (Dutton, 2004). In a cohort of 70 subjects with knee osteoarthritis, Hayes and colleagues found the majority of the subjects did not present with the typical capsular pattern of the knee (Hayes, Petersen, and Falconer, 1994).

A noncapsular pattern is a limitation in joint movement that does not follow the typical capsular pattern. Clinically, this loss of motion is caused by some other structure than the capsule, such as a bursa or torn meniscus.

Clinical Application of Joint Thrusts and Nonthrusts

Parameters applied to joint thrusts and nonthrusts vary widely. The force, frequency, and amplitude of techniques vary depending on client, clinician, and joint factors. For example, select clients may tolerate only small forces and amplitudes of nonthrusts over a short duration. If significant pain is present, nonthrusts should be applied using relatively small amplitudes and small forces. Maitland described four grades of nonthrust techniques (figure 2.1) (Maitland, 2005). Grades I and II are small and large amplitude nonthrusts, respectively, that do not reach the end of a joint's available arthrokinematic motion. These grades are generally for painful joints or apprehensive clients. Grades III and IV are large and small amplitude nonthrusts, respectively, that reach the end of a joint's available motion. These grades are generally used to increase arthrokinematic motion.

Recommendations for the force, frequency, and amplitude of nonthrust techniques also vary depending on the joint being treated. For example, in the lumbar spine, evidence shows the average force for grade IV nonthrusts ranges from 90 N to 240 N (Snodgrass, 2006). In the knee, grade IV nonthrusts appear to be between 30 N and 78 N (Pentelka, Hebron, Shapleski, and Goldshtein, 2012). In larger joints, such as the knee and hip, clinicians should be able to appreciate arthrokinematic motion visually in addition to feeling the joint translation with their hands. This observation is more challenging at smaller joints such as the cervical spine.

Concerning the frequency of nonthrusts, one estimate is that clinicians apply oscillations at a rate of 1 to 1.5 per second (Snodgrass, 2006). One recommendation has been made for at least 4 sets of 60 seconds of oscillations to induce the analgesia at the lumbar spine (Pentelka et al., 2012). However, clinicians should modify their frequency and duration of manual therapy techniques to fit client needs.

Safety and Risk of Injury

The clinician's intent to provide treatment to help a client with joint dysfunction may be overshadowed by possible risk of injury if the technique is not performed correctly or if the technique is not appropriate for the client. Clinical curriculums spend numerous hours on joint mobilization techniques in order to perfect technique and minimize injury. In the right hands, joint mobilization is very safe (Stevinson and Ernst, 2002).

One area of concern is spinal manipulation to the upper cervical spine. Although the incidence is low, manipulation to this anatomical region has repeatedly been associated with serious adverse events (Ernst, 2007). These manipulations are high-velocity rotatory techniques that can dissect the vertebral artery, resulting in stroke and possibly death.

Screening the client for contraindications and precautions will minimize injury. Also, informed consent should be granted by the client before joint mobilization/manipulation is performed.

Contraindications and Precautions for Thrust and Nonthrust Techniques

Clinicians must be vigilant in their assessment of clients to ensure they are appropriate for thrust or nonthrust maneuvers. The contraindications and precautions described here are not comprehensive of all contraindications and precautions for which clinicians should screen clients prior to manual therapy treatment.

Prior to performing thrusts or nonthrusts to the spine, clinicians should screen for the following red flags that may necessitate a medical referral: history of cancer, significant trauma, fractures, fever, steroid use, or unremitting pain. Other red flags specific to carotid artery disease or vertebral artery insufficiency include dizziness, drop attacks,

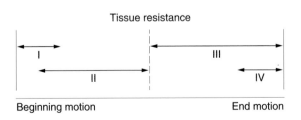

Figure 2.1 Maitland grades of movement.

Contraindications and Precautions for Thrust and Nonthrust Techniques

Contraindications

Bone tumor

Bone infection

Bone fracture

Bone dislocation

Osteomalacia, osteoporosis

Bone dysplasia or fusion

Recent surgery or surgical fusion

Long-term corticosteroid medication

Rheumatoid arthritis

Ligamentous rupture, instability

Acute myelopathy

Spinal cord compression

Cauda equine syndrome

Sudden vomiting, nausea, or vertigo

Vertebral basilar insufficiency

Carotid artery disease

Aortic aneurysm

Bleeding diatheses

Angina pectoris

Untreated cardiac insufficiency dysthymia

Acute abdominal pain

Lack of clinical examination or diagnosis

Lack of clinical skill

Lack of client consent

Precautions

Inflammatory joint process

Minor osteoporosis

Disc herniation or protrusion

Spondylolisthesis

Hypermobility or ligamentous laxity

Hypertension

Severe degenerative joint disease

Severe kyphosis or scoliosis

Systemic infections

Psychological dependence on techniques

Pain with a psychological overlay

---

dysphagia, dysarthria, diploplia, ataxia, numbness around the face, nausea, and nystagmus.

Thrusts should be avoided in areas of an unstable fracture, bone tumor, infectious disease, or osteomyelitis. Precautions for thrusts and nonthrusts should be taken in clients with osteoporosis, rheumatoid arthritis, disc pathology, spinal instability, or pregnancy. Also, if a client appears to be in poor health or fearful of the manual therapy technique, clinicians should adjust treatment accordingly to ensure safe treatment. Many contraindications and precautions for thrust and nonthrust techniques are listed in the accompanying sidebar (Puentedura and O'Grady, 2015).

Summary

General application guidelines for thrust and nonthrust techniques should be understood prior to client treatment. Subjective and objective examinations aid clinicians' choice of technique. Following the examinations, clinicians should have knowledge about the client's pathology as well as specific knowledge about the affected joint's arthrokinematics. Subsequent application of thrusts or nonthrusts can be applied using a variety of parameters. Clinicians should be mindful of the precautions, contraindications, and other safety concerns while performing the techniques in this text.

PART II

Mobilization and Manipulation of the Craniomandibular Complex and Spine

Part II consists of 4 chapters that cover thrust and nonthrust techniques for the temporomandibular joint (TMJ) and each region of the spine: cervical, thoracic, lumbar, and pelvic regions. Clinicians should be familiar with the information included in the introductory chapters, such as the general concepts and indications and contraindications for thrust and nonthrust techniques, when considering the use of techniques for the axial skeleton. Chapter 3 covers multiple nonthrust techniques for the frequently used TMJ. Thrust and nonthrust techniques for the cervical spine are presented in chapter 4. Given the anatomical differences in the cervical vertebrae, techniques specific to the upper and lower cervical spines are described. Chapter 5 covers the thoracic spine, including common thrust techniques to the vertebrae and techniques for the ribs. The final chapter of this section, chapter 6, covers lumbar spine and pelvic content. Many thrust and nonthrust techniques for the lumbar spine and sacrum are described in addition to those for the pubis and innominate.

Explicit instructions for all techniques are included with detailed overlaid photos to help the clinician with technique precision. The techniques described include multiple positions and potential modifications to accommodate clients who may have difficulty achieving one position or another. Current evidence for techniques is included in a table at the end of each chapter.

3

TEMPOROMANDIBULAR JOINT

LEARNING OBJECTIVES

After completing this chapter, you will be able to do the following:

◆ Identify the joint kinematics of the temporomandibular joint

◆ Describe appropriate positioning, movements, and intentions of temporomandibular joint mobilization techniques

◆ Cite evidence supporting temporomandibular joint mobilization techniques

The temporomandibular joint (TMJ)—or craniomandibular joint, as some call it—is a synovial joint articulation between the mandible and the temporal bone. The TMJ is likely the most frequently used joint in the human body. TMJ dysfunction can therefore be quite problematic, frustrating the simplest activities of daily living. Also, the function of the TMJ is closely related to that of the cervical spine and vice versa.

Anatomy

The mandible bone is suspended from the temporal bones on either side of the skull by ligaments (figure 3.1). Each TMJ is divided into an upper joint space and a lower joint space by the articular disc. The articular disc is a biconcave fibrocartilaginous structure occupying the space between the mandibular condyle and the mandibular articular fossa. Each joint space has a separate joint capsule

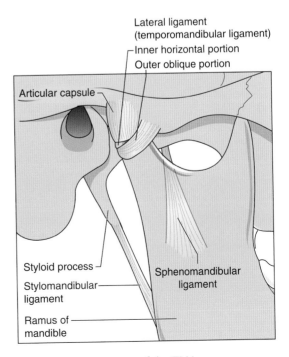

Figure 3.1 Ligaments of the TMJ.

with its own synovial lining. The lower joint is formed by the mandibular condyle and the inferior surface of the articular disc. The actual articulation with the temporal bone is indirect through the disc, and together with the articular disc and temporal bone form the TMJ. The lower joint space functions as a ginglymus (hinge) joint and an upper joint classified as an amphiarthrodial (plane) joint.

The lateral pterygoid muscle (figure 3.2) is the primary muscle responsible for jaw opening (mandibular protrusion), whereas the masseter and temporalis muscles (figure 3.3) are the primary muscles for jaw closing (mandibular retrusion). The masseter and temporalis muscles are also principal muscles of mastication.

Joint Kinematics

The function of the TMJ complex is unique in that movement in each of the joints is interdependent, simultaneous, and influenced significantly by each joint as well as by the occlusal surfaces of the teeth, cranium, and cervical spine. The arthrokinematics of the TMJ are complex because of the 3 degrees of freedom as well as the interdependent nature of the bicondylar joint structure. The motion in the lower joint space (articulation between the convex mandibular condyle and concave inferior surface of the articular disc) is primarily rotation.

The motion in the upper joint space (articulation between the concave superior surface of the articular disc and the concave inferior surface of the articular fossa) is primarily translation between the disc and the articular eminence. The possible movements of the mandible are depression (mouth opening), elevation (mouth closing), protrusion, retrusion, and lateral deviation to each side.

◆ *Mandibular depression* (mouth opening) is believed to occur in 2 phases, a rotation phase and a translation phase (figure 3.4a). With initial mouth opening, the condylar head rotates under the inferior surface of the articular disc (lower joint motion). This usually occurs in the first 35 to 50% of available opening. Once the capsular ligaments restrict further rotation of the mandibular head on the disc, the condyle and disc (condyle–disc complex) move together and translate anteriorly and inferiorly on the articular eminence (upper joint motion) to complete the final 50 to 65% of opening. Therefore, with mouth opening, an initial rotation motion in the lower joint is followed by a translation motion in the upper joint.

◆ *Mandibular elevation* (mouth closing) arthrokinematics occur in reverse order to mandibular depression—an initial translation motion in the upper joint is followed by a rotation motion in the lower joint.

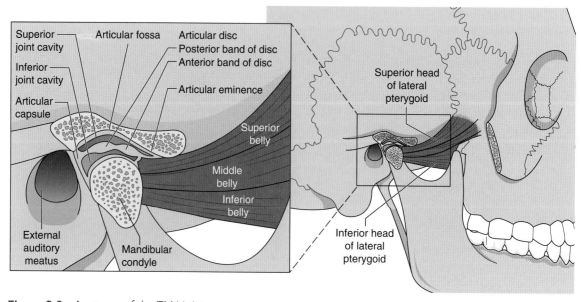

Figure 3.2 Anatomy of the TMJ joint.

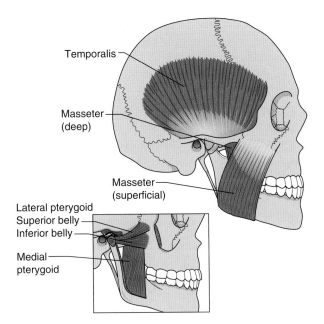

Temporalis

Masseter
(deep)

Masseter
(superficial)

Lateral pterygoid
Superior belly
Inferior belly

Medial
pterygoid

Figure 3.3 Muscles of the TMJ involved in mastication.

◆ *Mandibular protrusion* is the movement of sliding the mandible and lower teeth anteriorly relative to the maxilla and upper teeth (figure 3.4*b*). During protrusion, the condyle and disc translate anteriorly and slightly inferiorly until the complex abuts the articular eminence. Therefore, this motion is solely in the upper joint of the TMJ.

◆ *Mandibular retrusion* is the reverse of mandibular protrusion. It is the movement of the mandible and lower teeth sliding posteriorly relative to the maxilla and upper teeth (figure 3.4*c*). During this movement, the mandibular condyle and the articular disc translate posteriorly and increase the space between the anterior condyle–disc complex and the articular eminence. The posterior aspect of the complex approximates the posterior glenoid spine and compresses the soft tissue between the bony components of the posterior joint. Again, this motion is solely in the upper joint of the TMJ.

◆ *Lateral deviation/excursion* is the lateral movement of the mandible from side to side, sliding the lower teeth laterally relative to the upper teeth (figure 3.4*d*). The direction of lateral deviation is named for the side that the mandible is gliding toward. Lateral deviation/excursion occurs with small multiplanar movements because of the sloping of the articular eminence and happens primarily as a side-to-side translation. Lateral deviation/ excursion of the mandible is typically combined with slight rotations. This rotation most likely occurs in the upper portion of the joint because of the laxity of the joint capsule. Therefore, right lateral deviation is the movement of the mandible (and lower teeth) to the right of the maxilla (and upper teeth).

Clinical Tips

These tips apply to all intra-oral TMJ techniques:

- An important part of relaxing the client is to provide instruction on what the technique involves.
- Give the client frequent breaks to swallow.
- Prior to beginning the technique, the clinician and client should agree on signals to use during the technique. For example, a thumb-up sign indicates the client is doing fine; a thumb down indicates the technique is painful or that the client needs a break.
- Unless otherwise noted, the client's head should be kept in a neutral position.
- The clinician's gloves should remain clean throughout the technique.
- Ask the client about any latex allergies, dentures, loose teeth, or fillings.
- During all thrust and nonthrust techniques (for any joint), be sure to maintain visual observation of the client's reaction to the technique.

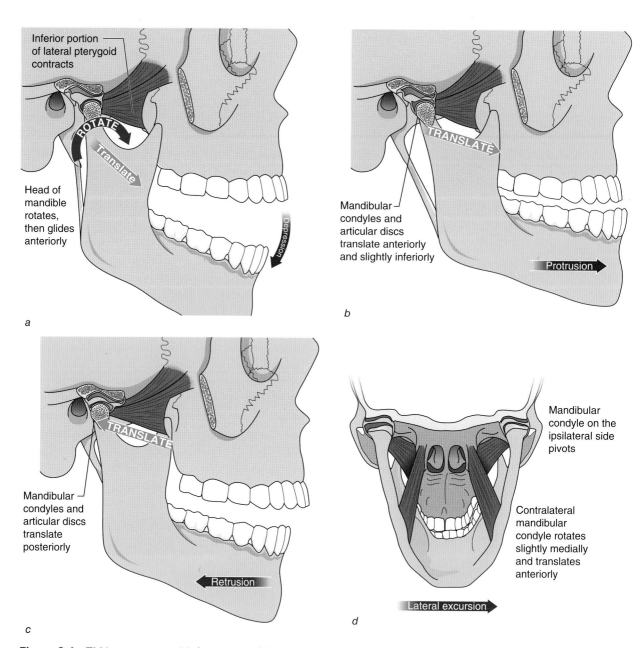

Figure 3.4 TMJ movements: (a) depression, (b) protrusion, (c) retrusion, and (d) lateral excursion.

TEMPOROMANDIBULAR JOINT ARTHROLOGY

Articular surfaces	Closed packed position	Resting position	Capsular pattern	ROM norms	End-feel
TMJ					
Lower joint Convex mandibular condyle articulating with concave inferior surface of articular disc **Upper joint** Concave superior surface of articular disc articulating with concave surface of articular fossa	Full occlusion	Teeth separated by 2–3 mm	Restriction in inferior glide	40- to 55-mm opening 3- to 6-mm protrusion 3- to 4-mm retrusion 10- to 12-mm lateral excursion	Soft tissue stretch for opening (mandibular depression) Bony during full occlusion of teeth (mouth closed/mandibular elevation Firm for protrusion and retrusion Capsular for lateral excursion

TMJ = temporomandibular joint; mm = millimeters

Inferior (Caudal) Glide

VIDEO 3.1 in the web study guide shows this technique.

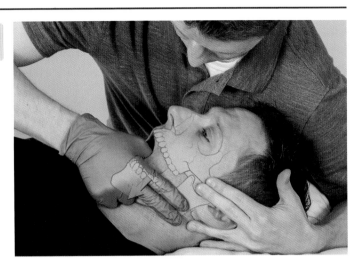

Client position: Supine on treatment table with arms and legs relaxed.

Clinician position: Standing at client's head facing client.

Stabilization: The position of the body on the treatment table serves as a stabilizing force; the clinician's cranial hand and deltopectoral groove stabilize the cranium.

Mobilization: Clinician's distal thumb is placed on the superior aspect of the posterior teeth and fingers along the lateral mandible. Distraction force is applied in a caudal direction primarily via the thumb. Force is low-velocity oscillations and/or sustained stretch.

Goal of technique: To help with multiplanar joint mobility limitations, pain with joint compression, pain with chewing, and general stiffness or capsular restriction. This mobilization is effective for increasing general TMJ motion.

Notes: The mobilization is most effective if the client can relax. Palpation of the TMJ joint can provide the clinician with feedback on the technique.

Anterior (Ventral) Glide

Client position: Supine on treatment table with arms and legs relaxed.

Clinician position: Standing at client's head facing client.

Stabilization: The position of the body on the treatment table serves as a stabilizing force; the clinician's cranial hand and deltopectoral groove stabilize the cranium.

Mobilization: Clinician's distal thumb is placed on the superior aspect of the posterior teeth and fingers along the lateral mandible. Distraction force is applied in a caudal-anterior direction primarily via the thumb. A slight initial caudal force is implemented prior to anteriorly directed force. Force is low-velocity oscillations and/or sustained stretch.

Goal of technique: To increase translation motion in the upper joint; beneficial for end-range mouth opening (mandibular depression), protrusion, and retrusion motions.

Notes: The mobilization is most effective if the client can relax. Palpation of the TMJ joint can provide the clinician with feedback on the technique.

Medial Glide

Client position: Supine on treatment table with arms and legs relaxed.

Clinician position: Standing at client's head facing client.

Stabilization: The clinician's cranial hand and deltopectoral groove stabilize the cranium.

Mobilization: Clinician's distal thumb is placed on the superior aspect of the posterior teeth, with the second and third fingers on lateral aspect of mandible with cranium stabilized. Distraction inferior followed by medial direction imparted primarily via second and third fingers

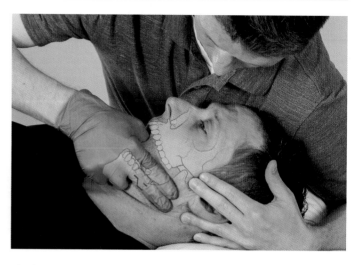

extra-orally (finger over finger placement if needed). Force is inferior distraction followed by medial glide of condyle. Force is low-velocity oscillations and/or sustained stretch.

Goal of technique: To increase medial/lateral joint mobility and lateral excursion movement.

Note: The primary force is through the second and third fingers so broad (and comfortable) finger purchase is necessary.

Lateral Glide

Client position: Supine on treatment table with arms and legs relaxed.

Clinician position: Standing at client's head facing client.

Stabilization: The clinician's cranial hand and deltopectoral groove stabilizes the cranium.

Mobilization: Clinician's cranial thumb is placed on the medial aspect of the mandible, with the second and third fingers of same hand placed on lateral aspect of mandible with cranium stabilized. Distraction inferior followed by lateral direction imparted primarily via

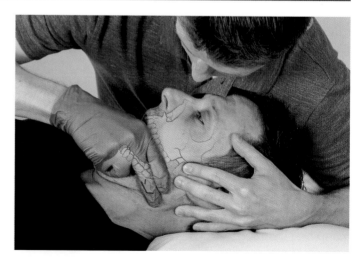

the thumb (on medial aspect of condyle) with stabilization from cranial hand. Force is inferior distraction followed by lateral glide of condyle. Force is low-velocity oscillations and/or sustained stretch.

Goal of technique: To increase medial/lateral joint mobility; particularly beneficial to increase contralateral lateral excursion motion.

Notes: The primary force is through the thumb, so broad (and comfortable) thumb purchase is necessary. Ensure that hand purchases are not unnecessarily uncomfortable.

Medial/Lateral Glide (Extra-Oral)

Client position: Supine on treatment table with arms and legs relaxed.

Clinician position: Standing at client's head (more cranial than inferior and anterior glides).

Stabilization: The position of the body on the treatment table serves as a stabilizing force; the clinician's cranial hand and deltopectoral groove stabilize the cranium.

Mobilization: Clinician's thenar eminence is purchased against the lateral mandible with the cranium stabilized. The thenar eminence imparts a medially directed force while the cranium is stabilized. Force

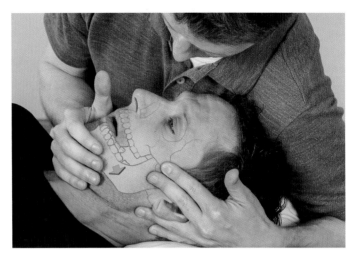

is medially directed (or relative lateral force on contralateral TMJ). Force is low-velocity oscillations and/or sustained stretch.

Goal of technique: To increase medial/lateral joint mobility; particularly beneficial to increase contralateral lateral excursion motion.

Notes: The primary force is the heel of the hand extra-orally, as described, so broad (and comfortable) heel of the hand purchase is necessary. Primary stabilization will be with clinician's deltopectoral groove and cranial hand. As always, broad hand purchase is advised for comfort.

Clinical tip: The clinician should be cautious of imparting an inferior distraction force if this is not warranted. Using the heel of the hand can encourage this inferior distraction. As with all mobilization/manipulation techniques, the clinician should monitor for immediate and latent response to treatment, modifying treatment accordingly.

Go to the web study guide and complete the case study for this chapter. The case study discusses a 50-year-old female with right-side jaw pain.

EVIDENCE FOR MANUAL THERAPY OF VARIOUS TEMPOROMANDIBULAR JOINT PATHOLOGIES

Study	Clients	Intervention and comparison (if any)	Outcome(s)
Utilization of thrust and nonthrust mobilization for various temporomandibular pathologies: Grade B			
Martins et al., 2016 (Level 1a)	8 studies (375 clients)	Musculoskeletal and osteopathic manipulative techniques versus various control groups	A significant difference ($p < 0.0001$) and large effect on active mouth opening and on pain during active mouth opening in favor of musculoskeletal manual techniques when compared to other conservative treatments for TMD.
Calixtre et al., 2015 (Level 1a)	8 studies	Myofascial release, soft tissue techniques, TMJ mobilizations, cervical and thoracic spine mobilizations versus various control groups	Moderate-to-high evidence that MT techniques are effective for pain and pain pressure threshold.
Armijo-Olivo et al., 2016 (Level 1a)	48 studies	Various MT treatment approaches versus various control groups	• MT targeted to the orofacial region in myogenous TMD: improved mouth opening and reduced jaw pain from baseline in all 3 groups; no superiority of intervention over control. • MT mobilization of the cervical spine and myogenous TMD: cervical spine mobilizations drastically decreased pain intensity and pain sensitivity immediately posttreatment. • MT plus jaw exercises in arthrogenous TMD: MT plus exercises significantly increased active mouth opening; symptoms and ROM compared to various controls. • MT and mixed TMD: mixed results for pain, mouth opening, and ROM across studies and treatment types. • MT plus exercises for mixed TMD: MT targeted to the orofacial region or in combination with cervical treatment was better than home exercises for the jaw and neck alone or treatment to cervical spine alone for improving mouth opening. Overall conclusion: MT alone or in combination with exercises at the jaw or cervical level showed promising effects. No high-quality evidence was found, indicating there is great uncertainty about the effectiveness of exercise and MT for treatment of TMD.
Crane et al., 2015 (Level 4)	1 subject with past medical history of head and neck lymphedema and temporomandibular dysfunction	Multimodal treatment plan, including complete decongestive therapy, MT, therapeutic exercise, and home program	Improved mandibular depression, decreased head and neck lymphedema, improved deep neck flexor endurance, decreased pain, and improved self-rated function.

MT = manual therapy; ROM = range of motion; TMD = temporomandibular disorder

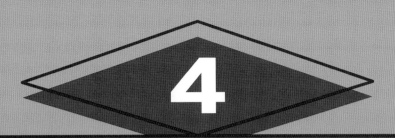

CERVICAL SPINE

CHAPTER OBJECTIVES

After completing this chapter, you will be able to do the following:

◆ Describe the joint kinematics of the various levels of the cervical spine

◆ Describe appropriate positioning, movements, and intentions of the various cervical spine joint mobilization techniques

◆ Identify evidence supporting cervical spine joint mobilization techniques

The cervical spine is a complex interaction of various anatomical structures and biomechanical movements. Movement of the cervical region of the spine is the greatest of any region of the spine, allowing for extensive visual ability, orientation in space, and daily tasks. As mentioned in chapter 3, a close mechanical and functional relationship exists between the cervical spine and the TMJ. The cervical spine also has a close functional and mechanical relationship with bilateral shoulders and the thoracic spine. Cervical spine–related pathology can, therefore, have quite complicating and deleterious effects.

Anatomy

The cervical spine consists of seven vertebrae and is divided into 4 anatomical units: the atlas, the axis, the C2-3 junction, and the rest of the cervical ver-

tebrae (figure 4.1). Functionally, the spine can be said to have 3 units: occipitoatlantal (C0-1) joint, atlantoaxial (C1-2) joint, and typical cervical spine (inferior facet of C2 through C7). As described in the following sections, the anatomical structure and function of each of these regions is unique and requires understanding when implementing the various treatment techniques. Assessment and subsequent treatment of the upper cervical spine (e.g., C0-1, C1-2, and C2-3) is unique to each level, as there are unique characteristics anatomically and functionally at each level. Assessment and treatment of the typical cervical spine (C2-7), on the other hand, is similar at each level (e.g., C3-4, C4-5) because of similar anatomy and arthrokinematic characteristics.

The specific detail of each of these 3 primary functional units of the cervical spine can be further described as follows:

◆ *Occipitoatlantal (C0-1) joint:* Some sources refer to this joint as the atlantooccipital joint. The C0-1 joint capsule and corresponding ligaments allow for motion due to their relatively lax status. The primary motion at this joint is a head-nodding motion. The amount of motion in this joint is greater in the sagittal plane than any other, yet relatively small compared with other cervical spine joints.

◆ *Atlantoaxial (C1-2) joint:* A primary function of the C1-2 joint is head rotation. Because of the amount of motion required at this joint, the capsule has a large amount of extensibility and is therefore relatively lax. It is typically held that greater than half of all cervical rotation is attributed to motion at this joint.

◆ *Typical cervical spine (C2-7):* Although these spinal levels have unique characteristics, similarities are shared among all levels (e.g., true spinous processes, zygoapophyseal [facet] joints with synovial capsules and intra-articular meniscoids, and intervertebral discs between each level). The joint capsules of the zygapophyseal joints are relatively lax and allow for a large range of motion (ROM).

The upper cervical spine ligaments are some of the most important of the human body because they provide necessary stability, including preventing the distraction of C1 on C2 and other check restraints. The primary cervical spine musculature serves not only to move the cervical spine, but to support the weight of the skull and to optimally position the sensory organs of the skull to respond to stimuli. The primary cervical spine flexors include the large sternocleidomastoid and scalene muscles (figure 4.2), although the deep cervical neck flexors (longus coli and longus capitis) are also important to flex the upper cervical spine with combined motions.

Joint Kinematics

The concept of coupled motion, or coupling, has been defined as "a phenomenon of consistent association of 1 motion (translation or rotation) about an axis with another motion about a second axis" (Blauvelt and Nelson, 1994). In other words, 1 motion cannot be produced without the other. Although this concept is traditionally accepted, scrutiny from recent literature reviews (Cook, 2003; Legaspi and Edmond, 2007) suggests using caution when applying the concepts of coupled motion to the evaluation and treatment of clients with spine pain. Coupling as traditionally accepted

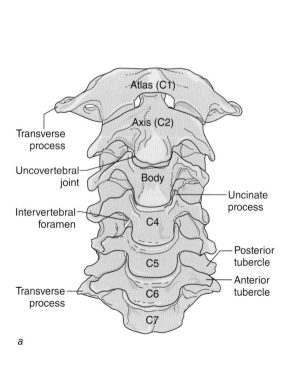

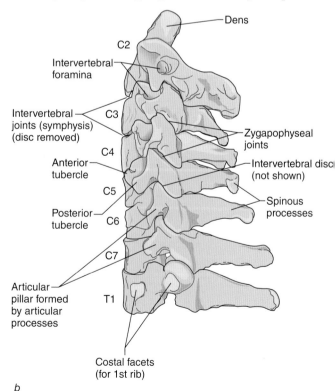

Figure 4.1 Cervical spine: *(a)* anterior view; *(b)* lateral view.

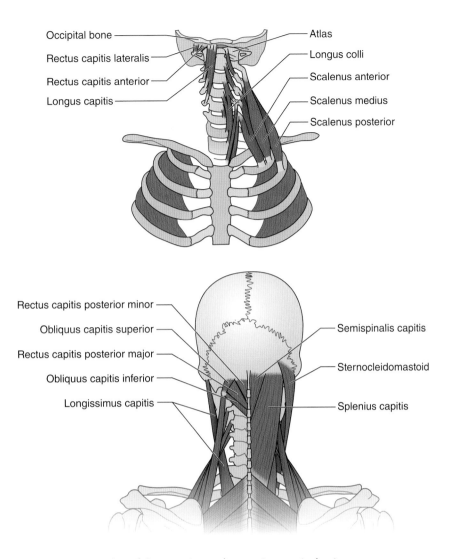

Figure 4.2 Muscles of the anterior and posterior cervical spine.

will be described here with this suggestion of caution in interpretation as well.

Occipitoatlantal (C0-1) Joint

The deep atlantal sockets of the atlas facilitate flexion/extension (or nodding) movements but impede other motions (Bogduk and Mercer, 2000). The nodding motion during flexion of the head is a result of rolling and gliding of the occipital condyles in their sockets (figure 4.3). As the head nods forward, the occipital condyles roll forward, rolling up the anterior wall of the atlantal socket. The flexor musculature, tension in the joint capsule, or both cause the occipital condyles to concomitantly translate downward and backward (Bogduk and Mercer, 2000). Therefore, forward nodding of the head (or anterior rotation of the occipital condyles)

is coupled with downward and posterior gliding of the condyles. During extension of the head on the atlas, the converse occurs. Lateral flexion, or sidebending, of the C0-1 joint involves a medial, inferior, and anterior directional glide of the ipsilateral occipital condyle with a corresponding lateral, posterior, and superior directional glide of the contralateral occipital condyle (figure 4.4).

Atlantoaxial (C1-2) Joint

Rotation, in the transverse plane (around a vertical axis), is the primary motion in the atlantoaxial (C1-2) joint. Since both articulating surfaces are convex, the apex of the cartilage on the inferior facet of C1 balances on the apex of the superior articular cartilage of C2 at rest. Axial rotation of C1 requires anterior displacement of 1 lateral mass and a reciprocal posterior displacement of the opposite lateral mass. The inferior articular cartilages of C1 must glide down the respective slopes of the convex superior articular cartilages of C2. Therefore, C1 essentially screws down onto C2 as it rotates (Koebke and Brade, 1982). A small amount of sidebending may accompany this rotation if the articular cartilages are asymmetrical. This coupling motion may be ipsilateral or contralateral depending on the bias of the asymmetry (White et al., 1975). The alar ligaments provide the principal restraint to axial rotation at this joint, with the lateral C1-2 joint capsule providing a minor role (Dvorak and Panjabi, 1987). The first 45° of rotation of the head on either side occurs at the C1-C2 level before initiation of movement of the lower cervical segments (Mercer and Bogduk, 2001).

Typical Cervical Spine (C2-7)

It has been suggested that the lower cervical spine demonstrates a consistent and predictable coupling pattern regardless of initiation of motion; sidebending and rotation occur to the same side (Panjabi, Oda, Crisco, Dvorak, and Grob, 1993; Panjabi and Crisco, 2001; Penning, 1978).

Flexion in the lower cervical spine, therefore, is always a combination of anterior translation and anterior rotation in the sagittal plane (with the inferior articular process of the superior ver-

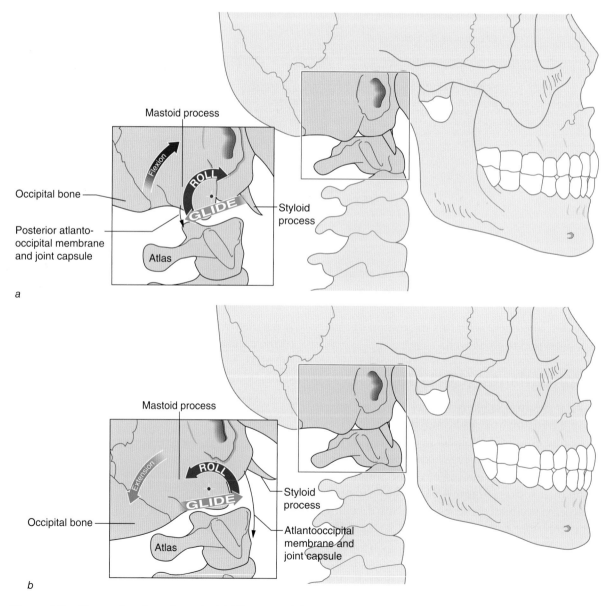

Figure 4.3 Kinematics of craniocervical (a) flexion and (b) extension at the atlantooccipital joint.

tebra gliding up the superior articular process of the vertebra below). *Extension* would therefore involve coupling of posterior sagittal rotation and posterior translation.

During axial *rotation*, the contralateral inferior articular process impacts the superior articular process of the inferior vertebra. Axial rotation continues only if the inferior articular process glides up the superior facet, resulting in ipsilateral sidebending of the moving superior vertebra. Therefore, rotation and sidebending of the lower cervical spine are always coupled ipsilaterally.

During sidebending, the ipsilateral inferior articular process moves down the slope of the superior articular process of the inferior vertebra (figure 4.5). The inferior articular process must then move posteriorly, resulting in the vertebra rotating toward the side of the sidebending. Therefore, again, sidebending and rotation of the lower cervical spine are always coupled ipsilaterally, regardless of which movement is initiated first.

Oversimplification of these motions is to suggest that with flexion the superior vertebra of the segment moves "up and forward" on the inferior

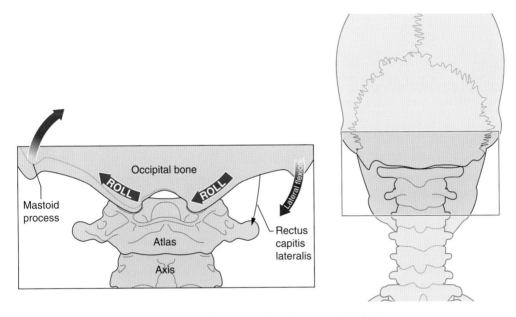

Figure 4.4 Kinematics of craniocervical lateral flexion at the atlantooccipital joint.

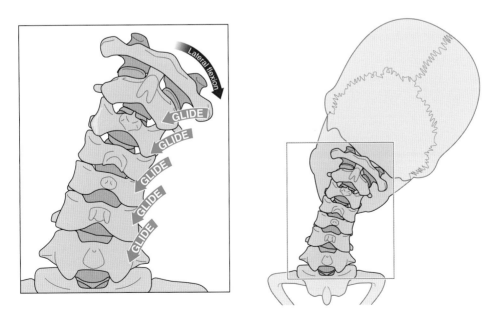

Figure 4.5 Kinematics of typical cervical spine (C2-7).

vertebra. Extension, therefore, would be a "down and back" motion of the superior vertebra on the inferior vertebra. Sidebending and rotation of the cervical spine would be ipsilateral extension (or down and back motion) and contralateral flexion (up and forward motion).

CERVICAL SPINE JOINT ARTHROLOGY

Articular surfaces	Closed packed position	Resting position	Capsular pattern	ROM norms	End-feel
OA joint (C0-1)					
C0 is convex C1 is concave	Not described	Not described	Extension and sidebending equally limited Rotation and flexion are not affected	Combined flexion and extension reported to range from 14–35° Sidebending reported to range from 2–11° Axial rotation reported to range from about 0–7°	Firm for all motions
Atlantoaxial Joint (C1-C2)					
Inferior surface of C1 is convex Superior surface of C2 is convex	Not described	Not described	Restriction with rotation	Flexion/extension is approximately 10° Rotation is approximately 40°	Firm for all motions
Typical cervical spine (C2-7 facet joints)					
Cranial facet is convex Caudal facet is concave	Full extension	Midway between flexion and extension	Sidebending and rotation are equally limited Extension is more limited than flexion	Flexion: 50° Extension: 60° Right sidebending: 45° Left sidebending: 45° Right rotation: 80° Left rotation: 80°	Firm for all motions

Seated Distraction

Client position: Seated with arms relaxed. For increased comfort, client may recline against a pillow placed between client and clinician.

Clinician position: Standing behind client with hands cupped below each side of the occiput, with the thenar eminences contacting the mastoid processes and client's back against clinician's chest (female clinicians can use a pillow barrier) and elbows in front of client's bilateral shoulders to provide appropriate angle of distraction.

Stabilization: Client's body serves as stabilization.

Mobilization: As client inhales, slightly lift the skull superiorly or simply stabilize the skull. Maintain the upward directed force as client exhales and descends.

Goal of technique: General distraction of the cervical spine.

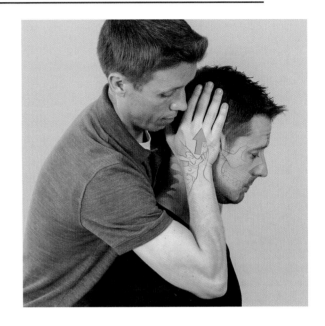

Notes: Increasing the amount of cervical spine flexion will generally target lower cervical spine segments. To maintain mechanical advantage, keep elbows as close together as possible. Additionally, lifting with your body (e.g., starting with knees bent) is advised for larger clients or clients that require more distraction.

Supine Distraction

Client position: Supine with arms relaxed.

Clinician position: Standing or sitting at the head of treatment table, facing client.

Stabilization: Client's body on treatment table serves as stabilization, in addition to the delto-pectoral groove of the clinician on the client's forehead, which limits flexion of the neck. A stabilizing hand can be used at any lower segment to aid localization of the technique.

Mobilization: Grasping the occiput with 1 hand, with OA joint in slight extension, a cephalic force is applied to the cervical spine.

Goal of technique: General distraction of the cervical spine.

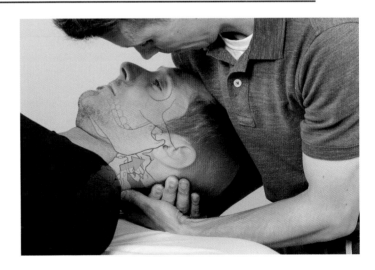

Notes: Varying degrees of flexion can be applied, depending on symptom relief. A towel can be used for mobilization in place of the hands. If using a towel, keep it close to sides of client's face to ensure it does not slip off.

Upper Cervical Distraction

Client position: Supine with head relaxed.

Clinician position: Sitting next to client's head with mobilizing forearm supinated beneath the occiput, and stabilizing hand beneath chin.

Stabilization: Two fingers beneath the mandible prevents OA joint flexion during the distraction maneuver.

Mobilization: Apply traction to the upper cervical spine by pronating the mobilizing forearm cephalically, contacting the radius onto the external occipital protuberance (ensuring a comfortable purchase for both the client and clinician).

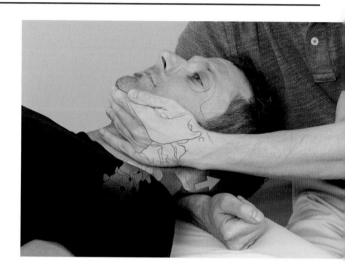

Goal of technique: General distraction of the cervical spine.

Notes: This technique might help relieve headaches. A towel can be placed beneath the forearm to limit cervical extension. The majority of the force should come from the purchase on the external occipital protuberance, and not on the mandible (especially for clients with temporomandibular joint dysfunction).

Unilateral Occipitoatlantal (C0-1) Distraction

VIDEO 4.1 **in the web study guide shows this technique.**

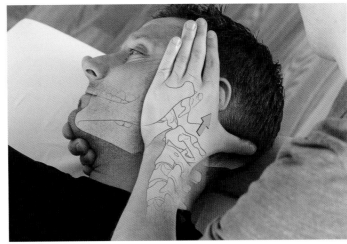

Client position: Supine with head rotated away from the side to be mobilized.

Clinician position: Standing at head of treatment table with nonmobilizing hand beneath client's chin and nonmobilizing forearm cradling client's head (a chin cradle grip).

Stabilization: The client's body serves as stabilization, as does the nonmobilizing hand beneath the client's mandible.

Mobilization: Using the heel of the hand to purchase the inferior portion of the mastoid process, the clinician mobilizes the occiput superiorly.

Goal of technique: To treat an OA joint restriction, regardless of restriction type. As with all distraction techniques, this is a general technique for restricted motion of the joint. If the goal is to facilitate OA joint flexion, the hand on the chin should allow the chin to move caudally (OA flexion).

Notes: The clinician's mobilizing arm's forearm is best positioned along the client's deltopectoral groove for accurate direction of mobilization. This may not be an appropriate technique for a client with temporomandibular joint dysfunction because of the pressure on the joint via contact on the mandible.

Clinical Tip

Temporomandibular joint dysfunction has been shown to correlate with cervical spine–related dysfunction in some clients. With any cervical spine mobilization technique involving purchase on the mandible, the clinician must be cognizant of clients with potential temporomandibular joint dysfunction. It may be unwarranted to provide much force to the mandible in these clients to prevent worsening of potential temporomandibular symptoms.

Occipitoatlantal (C0-1) Flexion

 VIDEO 4.2 in the web study guide shows this technique.

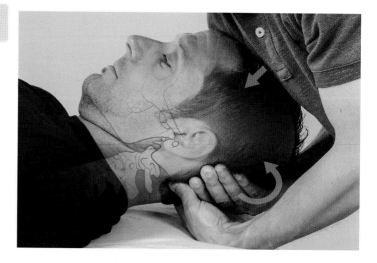

Client position: Supine with head at top of treatment table.

Clinician position: Standing at head of treatment table facing client, cupping the occiput with 1 hand with the head in slight flexion, and the thumb and index finger of the other hand on the lamina of the atlas (C1).

Stabilization: The hand on the atlas (C1) stabilizes, as does the clinician's delto-pectoral groove on the client's forehead.

Mobilization: The hand cradling the client's occiput provides flexion roll of the occiput on the atlas while the clinician's delto-pectoral groove mobilizes the head in an anterior-to-posterior direction. The combined actions create OA joint flexion.

Goal of technique: To treat an OA joint flexion (nodding) restriction; nonspecifically, for a unilateral OA joint flexion restriction.

Notes: The head can be rotated to either side to bias either OA joint articulation. This technique can create a pressure sensation in the throat in some clients. As with all techniques, continuously monitor the client's response.

Prone Occipitoatlantal (C0-1) Posterior to Anterior Glide

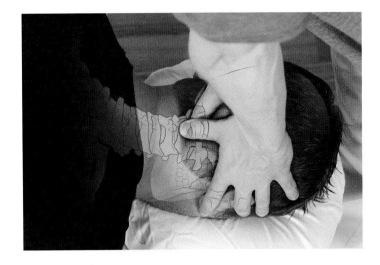

Client position: Prone with arms relaxed at side, head neutral.

Clinician position: Standing at head of treatment table facing client.

Stabilization: Client's body weight on the treatment table serves as stabilization.

Mobilization: Clinician palpates the suboccipital region and uses thumb-over-thumb contact over the OA joint. Push the paraspinal musculature medially to avoid compressing through tissue when performing this assessment. Light pressure only is applied initially in the direction of the client's orbit (eye). If tolerated well, repeat movements and reassess.

Goal of technique: To treat a unilateral OA joint restriction or pain with a technique that responds favorably to repeated mobilizations.

Notes: The mobilization is most effective when the clinician ensures the proper angle (toward the client's ipsilateral eye). Therefore, the client will have to lean the upper body slightly toward the client's feet and keep bilateral elbows straight. Because the clinician's center of mass is leaning forward, the clinician should not increase pressure on the purchase points on the client.

Clinical Tip

With all prone spine mobilizations (cervical, thoracic, and lumbar), the clinician must do the following:

- Properly take up the soft tissue slack and purchase the joint to be treated.
- Perform a purchase that is comfortable for both client and clinician.
- Properly assess the amount of joint play at the segment to be assessed.
- Properly assess the end-feel and client response.
- Choose the appropriate grade of mobilization/manipulation to best treat the client.
- Perform reassessment throughout treatment, after treatment session, and between treatment sessions.

Supine Atlantoaxial (C1-2) Rotation

Client position: Supine with head at top of treatment table.

Clinician position: Standing at head of treatment table facing client.

Stabilization: Client's bodyweight on the treatment table provides adequate stabilization. Clinician places distal interphalangeal joint of index finger of mobilizing hand on the posterior-lateral aspect of C2 (axis) and places palm on the occiput.

Mobilization: Clinician places mobilizing index finger along the length of C1 (atlas). Clinician then sidebends the head maximally in the contralateral direction of rotation to be treated. While maintaining sidebending, clinician mobilizes C1 (atlas) on C2 (axis) in direction of restriction.

Goal of technique: To treat a C1-2 joint restriction or pain with a technique that responds favorably to repeated mobilizations.

Notes: The treatment plane is essentially horizontal given the orientation of the C1-C2 articulations. Be sure to maintain sidebending during rotation and to avoid placing mobilizing thumb on client's throat.

Seated Atlantoaxial (C1-2) Rotation

 VIDEO 4.3 **in the web study guide shows this technique.**

Client position: Sitting upright.

Clinician position: Standing behind client.

Stabilization: No stabilizing force is needed.

Mobilization: Using thumb-over-thumb or single-thumb placement over the posterior portion of lateral C1 transverse process, the clinician mobilizes the process anteriorly as the client rotates to the desired contralateral direction. The thumb(s) should maintain contact with C1's transverse process as the client actively rotates head in the contralateral direction (left purchase and right cervical rotation, vice versa) and returns to midline.

Goal of technique: To treat a C1-2 joint restriction or pain with a technique that responds favorably to repeated mobilizations.

Notes: The treatment plane is essentially horizontal given the orientation of the C1-C2 articulations. Do not push the client's head and cervical spine into flexion. Client maintains an upright cervical spine posture. Take care not to grasp the client's throat.

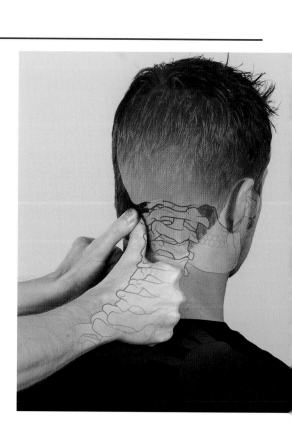

Prone Atlantoaxial (C1-2) Posterior to Anterior Glide

Client position: Prone with arms relaxed at side; head in neutral starting position.

Clinician position: Standing at head of treatment table facing client.

Stabilization: Client's body weight on the treatment table serves as stabilization.

Mobilization: Clinician palpates facet joint of C2-3 with thumb-over-thumb contact over the joint. Clinician passively rotates client's head to the ipsilateral side (approximately 30°). Light pressure only is applied initially in the direction of the mouth. If tolerated well, repeat movements and reassess.

Goal of technique: To treat a unilateral C1-2 joint restriction or pain with a technique that responds favorably to repeated mobilizations.

Notes: The mobilization is most effective when the clinician ensures the proper angle (toward the client's mouth). Therefore, the client will have to step to the client's opposite shoulder and lean a little toward the client's feet with the upper body and ensure to keep bilateral elbows straight. Again, the clinician should be cognizant of not increasing pressure to the purchase on the client.

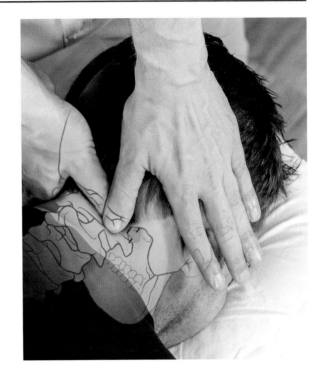

Prone C2-3 Posterior to Anterior Glide

Client position: Prone with arms relaxed at side, head neutral.

Clinician position: Standing at head of treatment table facing client.

Stabilization: Client's body weight on the treatment table serves as stabilization.

Mobilization: Clinician palpates facet joint of C2-3 with thumb-over-thumb contact over the joint. Light pressure only is applied initially in the direction of the table. If tolerated well, repeat movements and reassess.

Goal of technique: To treat a unilateral C2-3 joint restriction or pain with a technique that responds favorably to repeated mobilizations.

Notes: The mobilization is most effective when the clinician ensures the proper angle (toward the client's mouth). Therefore, the client will have to lean over slightly (but not to the extent for the C0-1 PA glide previously described).

Cervical Flexion

Client position: Supine with head at top of treatment table.

Clinician position: Standing or sitting at head of treatment table facing client, cupping the occiput and segment to be mobilized with 1 hand; the thumb and index finger of the other hand is around the inferior segment's spinous process.

Stabilization: The hand grasping the inferior segment's spinous process serves to stabilize, as does the clinician's deltopectoral groove on the client's forehead.

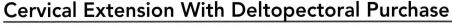

Mobilization: The mobilizing hand grasps the spinous process of the segment to be mobilized and draws it up and forward in attempts of replicating normal flexion arthrokinematics.

Goal of technique: To treat a flexion (up and forward) joint restriction or pain with a technique that responds favorably to repeated mobilizations.

Note: The mobilization is most effective if the neck is flexed up to the segment to be mobilized.

Cervical Extension With Deltopectoral Purchase

Client position: Supine with head at top of treatment table.

Clinician position: Standing or sitting at head of treatment table facing client, cupping the occiput and segment to be mobilized with 1 hand; the thumb and index finger of the other hand is around the inferior segment's spinous process.

Stabilization: The hand grasping the inferior segment's spinous process serves to stabilize, as does the clinician's deltopectoral groove on the client's forehead.

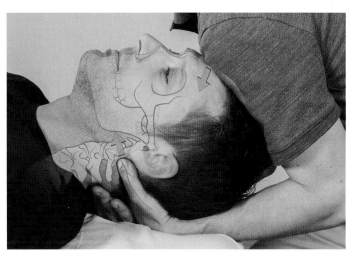

Mobilization: The mobilization is performed primarily via pressure from the deltopectoral groove through the forehead, with concomitant stabilization of the inferior segment's spinous process. The mobilizing hand may also assist the spinous process of the segment to be mobilized down and back.

Goal of technique: To treat an extension (down and back) joint restriction or pain with a technique that responds favorably to repeated mobilizations.

Note: The mobilization is most effective if the neck is extended down to the segment to be mobilized.

Cervical Extension

Client position: Supine with head at top of treatment table.

Clinician position: Standing at head of treatment table facing client.

Stabilization: Client's bodyweight on the treatment table provides adequate stabilization.

Mobilization: Clinician first ensures that client's neck is in neutral. Because clients will often present in extension when lying supine, a towel or firm surface may need to be placed under the occiput to promote neutral spine posture. Place the radial boarder of the index fingers along the lamina of the vertebra to be mobilized. Lift ventrally with both fingers until extension occurs at the desired segment.

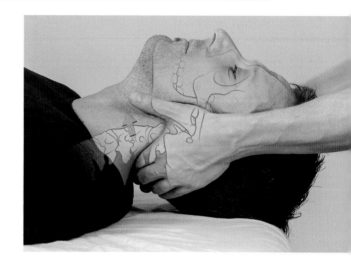

Goal of technique: To treat an extension joint restriction or pain with a technique that responds favorably to repeated mobilizations.

Note: The mobilization is most effective in treating an extension (down and back) joint restriction or pain.

Unilateral Down and Back

 VIDEO 4.4 **in the web study guide shows this technique.**

Client position: Supine with head at top of treatment table.

Clinician position: Standing at head of treatment table facing client.

Stabilization: The stabilizing hand cradles client's skull.

Mobilization: Client's head should be sideglided up to the segment to be mobilized (contralateral to the side of the mobilizing hand). The radial aspect of the clinician's mobilizing hand's metacarpophalangeal joint of the index finger

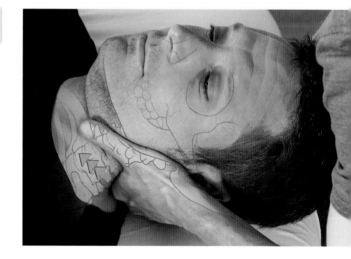

should be placed on the posterior-lateral aspect of the segment to be mobilized. The mobilization should be in a down and back direction, as if sliding the mobilizing hand down and around a cylinder toward the client's contralateral shoulder.

Goal of technique: To facilitate the down and back (closing/extension) motion on the ipsilateral side.

Notes: The cervical spine can also be extended, sidebent, and rotated to the level being mobilized in attempts to isolate the segment to be treated. If necessary, this technique can be used as indirect mobilization to facilitate contralateral motion up and forward.

Unilateral Down and Back Grade V (Downslope Thrust)

Client position: Supine with head at top of treatment table.

Clinician position: Standing at head of treatment table facing client.

Stabilization: Client's head resting on treatment table serves as stabilization.

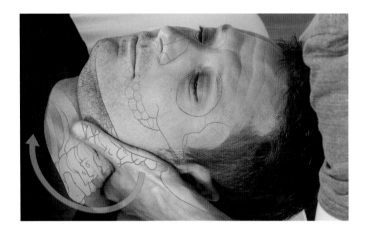

Mobilization: The radial aspect of the bilateral hand's metacarpophalangeal joint of the index finger should be placed on the posterior-lateral aspect of the segment to be mobilized. Target the level to be treated (left side cervical spine in photo) with bilateral extension, up and forward at that level on left (sidebending right in photo), and rotate in direction of restriction (left in photo). In other words, the setup is as follows: bilateral extension, contralateral sidebending, and ipsilateral rotation. The technique should be in a down and backward direction toward the contralateral shoulder, as if moving the hand down and around a cylinder.

Goal of technique: To facilitate the down and back (closing/extension) motion on the ipsilateral side.

Notes: This technique can be used as indirect mobilization to facilitate contralateral motion up and forward. The rotation thrust amplitude should be small.

Unilateral Up and Forward

> **VIDEO 4.5 in the web study guide shows this technique.**

Client position: Supine with head at top of treatment table.

Clinician position: Standing at head of treatment table facing client.

Stabilization: The radial aspect of the stabilizing hand's index finger is placed posterior to the inferior segment's transverse process. The articular pillar and spinous process rest along this index finger.

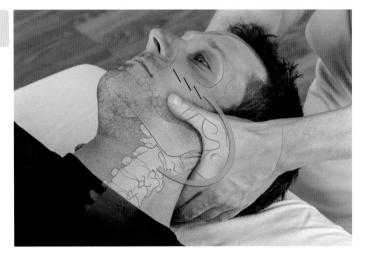

Mobilization: The radial aspect of the mobilizing hand's proximal interphalangeal joint of the index finger should be placed on the posterior-lateral aspect of the segment to be mobilized. The mobilization should be in an up and forward direction toward the contralateral eye, as if moving the hand up and around a cylinder.

Goal of technique: To facilitate the up and forward (opening/flexion) motion on the ipsilateral side.

Notes: The cervical spine can also be flexed, sidebent away, and rotated away to the level being mobilized. The head can be placed on the clinician's abdomen to facilitate relaxation. This technique can be used as indirect mobilization to facilitate contralateral motion down and back.

Unilateral Up and Forward Grade V (Upslope Thrust)

Client position: Supine with head at top of treatment table.

Clinician position: Standing at head of treatment table facing client.

Stabilization: Client's head resting on table serves as stabilization.

Mobilization: Bilateral hands are used in this technique. The radial aspect of the bilateral hand's proximal interphalangeal joint of the index finger should be placed on the posterior-lateral aspect of the segment to be mobilized. Target the level to be treated (left side cervical spine in photo) with bilateral flexion, down and

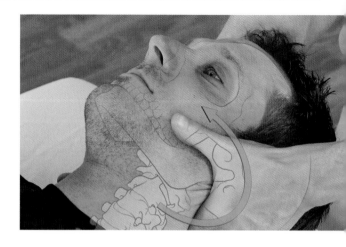

back at that level on left (sidebending left in photo), and rotate in direction of restriction (right rotation in photo). In other words, the setup is as follows: bilateral flexion, ipsilateral sidebending, and contralateral rotation. The technique should be in an up and forward direction toward the contralateral eye, as if moving the hand up and around a cylinder.

Goal of technique: To facilitate the up and forward (opening/flexion) motion on the ipsilateral side.

Notes: Skilled clinicians can use notes from previous technique regarding use of the abdomen. As with all thrust techniques, the rotation thrust amplitude should be small.

Central Posterior to Anterior Glides

Client position: Prone with head in neutral.

Clinician position: Standing at head of treatment table facing client.

Stabilization: The client's head in the treatment table opening provides stabilization.

Mobilization: With index fingers positioned as shown, push bilateral paraspinal muscles toward midline to decrease soft tissue tension in the area. The clinician palpates the spinous process of the level to be treated with thumb-over-thumb contact over the joint. Light pressure only is applied initially in the direction of the table. If tolerated well, repeat movements and reassess. Multiple hand positions may be used to mobilize

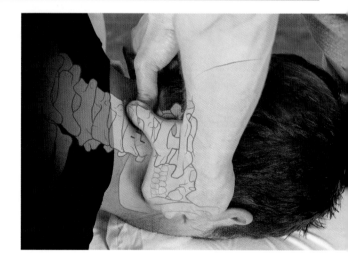

the target segment's spinous process anteriorly. For example, thumb over thumb, thumb by thumb, or a pincer grip may all be used over the target segment.

Goal of technique: To treat a joint restriction or pain with a technique that responds favorably to repeated mobilizations.

Notes: Lowering the head of the table (increasing cervical spine flexion) may facilitate palpation of the lower cervical segments. Again, the client should lean the upper body over segments being assessed without increasing pressure on client.

Unilateral Posterior to Anterior

Client position: Prone with head in neutral.

Clinician position: Standing at head of treatment table facing client.

Stabilization: Client's head in the table opening provides stabilization.

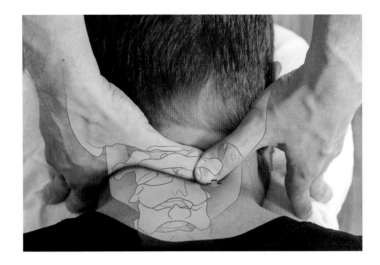

Mobilization: Clinician palpates the facet joint of the segment and side to be treated with thumb-over-thumb contact over the joint. Light pressure only is applied initially in the direction of the table. If tolerated well, repeat movements and reassess. Multiple hand positions may be used to mobilize the target segment's transverse process anteriorly. For example, thumb over thumb or thumb by thumb can be used over the target segment.

Goal of technique: To treat a unilateral joint restriction or pain with a technique that responds favorably to repeated mobilizations.

Notes: Lowering the head of the table (increasing cervical spine flexion) may facilitate palpation of the lower cervical segments. Pushing the tissue toward or away from midline can decrease the soft tissue tension at the level to be treated.

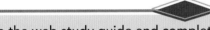

Go to the web study guide and complete the case study for this chapter. The case study discusses a 24-year-old physical therapy student complaining of headaches.

EVIDENCE FOR MANUAL THERAPY OF VARIOUS
CERVICAL SPINE PATHOLOGIES

Study	Clients	Intervention and comparison (if any)	Outcome(s)
Utilization of thrust and nonthrust mobilization for neck pain with mobility deficits			
Acute neck pain with mobility deficits: Grade B (thoracic manipulation, neck ROM, and strengthening of shoulder girdle) Grade C (cervical manipulation and/or mobilization)			
Blanpied et al., 2016	Level 3 (8 studies)	Thoracic spine manipulation compared to various groups	Effective for reducing pain over the immediate and short term. This finding was consistent over the intermediate term, but the magnitude of effect was small for pain, function, and quality of life in acute and chronic neck pain clients.
	Level 5 (2 studies)	Cervical manipulation	1 to 4 sessions of a single cervical manipulation for reducing pain over the immediate but not short term in acute and chronic neck pain clients.
	Level 4 (1 study)	Cervical manipulation as stand-alone therapy	Conflicting evidence supporting the use of multiple sessions of cervical manipulation as a stand-alone therapy in acute and chronic neck pain clients.
	Level 2 (5 studies)	Cervical manipulation compared to cervical mobilization	No benefit of manipulation when compared to mobilization for reducing pain and improving function, quality of life, global perceived effect, and patient satisfaction over the immediate, short, and intermediate term in acute and chronic neck pain clients.
	Level 4 (2 studies)	Cervical mobilization and ipsilateral manipulation compared to control	Benefit in using cervical mobilization and ipsilateral manipulation for reducing pain over the immediate term in clients with acute and subacute neck pain.
	Level 3 (2 studies)	Cervical manipulation compared to oral medication combinations	Benefit for multiple sessions of cervical manipulation for reducing pain and improving function over the long term in clients with acute and subacute neck pain.
	Level 3 (1 study)	Cervical manipulation or mobilization alone	Benefit of combination of manual therapy for providing analgesic benefits over the short term in acute and subacute neck pain clients.

Study	Clients	Intervention and comparison (if any)	Outcome(s)
Subacute neck pain with mobility deficits: Grade C (thoracic manipulation and cervical manipulation and/or mobilization)			
Blanpied et al., 2016	Level 4 (3 studies)	Single session of thoracic manipulation control	Reduced pain, improved ROM over short term, reduced disability in mid-term with single session of thoracic manipulation.
	Level 3 (1 study) Level 4 (1 study)	Single session of (a) cervical (1 level 4 study) and (b) thoracic (1 level 3 study) manipulation compared to control	No benefit for either cervical or thoracic manipulation reduced pain in immediate term.
	Level 3 (1 study)	Cervical manipulation compared to cervical mobilization	Benefit of both; no difference between groups after 2 weeks of treatment on improving function or reducing pain, disability, or days to perceived recovery.
	Level 3 (1 study)	Cervical manipulation alone or with advice and home program compared to cervical mobilization and strengthening exercises	Benefit of both; no benefit of 1 group over other for reducing pain and disability in short or long term.
	Level 4 (1 study)	Cervical mobilization compared to usual care	No benefit of cervical mobilization compared to usual care for reducing pain over intermediate term.
Chronic neck pain with mobility deficits: Grade B (thoracic manipulation and cervical manipulation or mobilization, deep neck flexor strengthening, and scapulothoracic stretching/strengthening/neuromuscular exercise)			
Blanpied et al., 2016	Level 3 (3 studies)	Single session of thoracic manipulation compared to control	Benefit for single session of thoracic manipulation for pain in the immediate term.
	Level 4 (8 studies)	Single session of supine thoracic manipulation compared to control	Benefit for single session of thoracic manipulation for pain in the immediate term.
	Level 4 (1 study)	Upper thoracic compared to cervical manipulation	Benefit of upper thoracic manipulation for reducing pain in immediate term.
	Level 4 (1 study)	12 sessions over 4 weeks of anterior-posterior unilateral accessory procedures compared to rotational or transverse accessory procedures	Benefit of anterior-posterior procedures for immediate-term pain relief.
	Level 3 (2 studies)	Cervical manipulation compared to medication	No benefit of cervical manipulation for reducing pain in immediate term.
	Level 4 (1 study)	Cervical mobilization compared to exercise, laser, pulsed ultrasound, acupuncture, massage	No benefit of cervical mobilization for mediate- to mid-term improvement in quality of life.

(continued)

EVIDENCE FOR MANUAL THERAPY OF VARIOUS
CERVICAL SPINE PATHOLOGIES *(continued)*

Study	Clients	Intervention and comparison (if any)	Outcome(s)
Utilization of thrust and nonthrust mobilization for chronic neck pain with WAD: Grade B			
Blanpied et al., 2016 (Level 3)	1 study	Mobilization or manipulation	Benefit of mobilization or manipulation and a multimodal approach for symptom and function related to WAD.
Utilization of thrust and nonthrust mobilization for neck pain and associated disorder: Grade C			
Wong et al., 2015 (Level 1a)	15 studies	Cervical and thoracic manipulation compared to high-dose supervised home exercises	Cervical and thoracic manipulation provides no additional benefit to high-dose supervised exercises.
Utilization of thrust and nonthrust mobilization for neck pain with headache			
Subacute neck pain with headache: Grade B			
Blanpied et al., 2016 (Level 3)	4 studies	Cervical manipulation and mobilization compared to control	Benefit in reducing headache intensity and frequency over immediate through long term.
Chronic neck pain with headache: Grade B			
Blanpied et al., 2016 (Level 3)	4 studies	Cervical manipulation and mobilization compared to exercise alone or manipulation plus exercise	Small to no benefit in using cervical manipulation for reducing headache pain and frequency over short term.

ROM = range of motion; WAD = whiplash associated disorder

5

THORACIC SPINE

LEARNING OBJECTIVES

After completing this chapter, you will be able to do the following:

◆ Identify the joint kinematics of the thoracic spine

◆ Describe appropriate positioning, movements, and intentions for thoracic spine joint mobilization techniques

◆ Identify evidence supporting thoracic spine joint mobilization techniques

The thoracic spine is a unique section of joints, especially given its relationship to the ribs and thick trunk musculature. The thoracic spine contains more articulations than the adjacent cervical or lumbar sections of the spine, with most thoracic vertebrae exhibiting 12 sites of articulation. Despite this abundance of articulations, the thoracic spine is stiffer and less mobile than the rest of the spine. The ribs, serving to protect the viscera, demand a stable base. Moreover, the energy transfer from the lower extremities to the upper extremities and vice versa requires a thorax capable of transferring large forces.

Anatomy

The thoracic spine is composed of 12 vertebrae. Most of these 12 vertebrae have 12 articulations: 4 zygapophyseal or facet articulations, 2 costotransverse, 4 costovertebral, and 2 with the intervertebral discs above and below (figure 5.1). The vertebral bodies of the thoracic spine are taller posteriorly than anteriorly, resulting in the thoracic spine's posterior convexity. The apex of this kyphotic curve is at the seventh or eighth thoracic vertebra. Vertebral discs exist between each thoracic segment, which aid in shock absorption and facilitation of thoracic motion. The spinous processes of the thoracic spine are generally parallel to the transverse processes of the segment below.

The facet joints of the thoracic spine are formed by a taut capsule surrounding the superior and inferior articular processes of adjacent vertebrae. The articulating surfaces of the thoracic spine facet joints demonstrate significant variability from the upper thoracic region to the lower thoracic region. The upper region's joints demonstrate strong resemblance to the cervical spine, while the lower region's joints show similarities to the lumbar spine, favoring sagittal plane motion. The superior articular processes generally face posteriorly (about 60 to 80° from the horizontal plane) and slightly superiorly, while the inferior articular processes face anteriorly and slightly inferiorly.

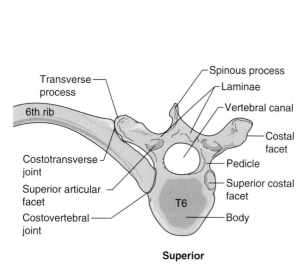

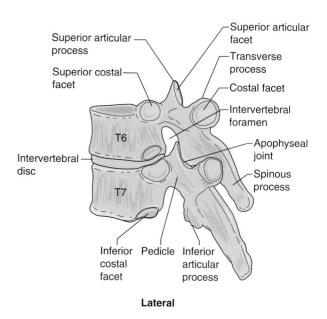

Figure 5.1 Thoracic spine joints.

The soft tissues supporting the thoracic spine are numerous. The anterior and posterior longitudinal ligaments, ligamentum flavum, interspinous ligaments, and supraspinous ligament provide sagittal plane support (figure 5.2). The ribs, with their corresponding capsules and ligaments as well as the intertransverse ligaments, support the thoracic spine in the frontal and transverse planes. The primary muscles surrounding the thoracic spine and ribs include the erector spinae, latissimus dorsi, trapezius, serratus, and rhomboids posteriorly; and the obliques and pectoralis muscles anteriorly. Intercostal muscles and an abundance of other respiratory muscles provide additional strength around the thoracic spine (figure 5.3).

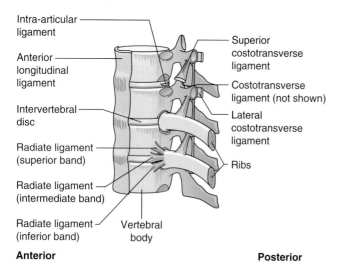

Figure 5.2 Ligament support of the costovertebral joint.

Joint Kinematics

To describe the joint kinematics of the thoracic spine, the motion of the superior vertebrae's articular processes on the inferior vertebrae's articular processes will be detailed (e.g., T4 on T5). During thoracic spine flexion, the inferior articular facets of the superior vertebrae (e.g., T4) move superiorly and anteriorly (up and forward) on the superior articular facets of the inferior vertebrae (e.g., T5). Thoracic spine extension involves opposite motions, as the uppermost facets glide inferiorly and posteriorly (down and back) on the lowermost facets (figure 5.4). Sidebending is a result of the ipsilateral articular processes gliding inferiorly, while the contralateral articular processes glide superiorly. This motion is limited in the thoracic spine by rib approximation ipsilaterally and contralateral soft tissues being stretched. Concerning rotation, the coupling arthrokinematics of the thoracic spine are inconsistent in the literature.

During thoracic spine extension and inspiration, inferior gliding of the rib at the costotransverse joint typically occurs. Simultaneously, the ribs will typically rotate posteriorly, meaning the anterior aspect of the rib travels superiorly, while the posterior aspect travels inferiorly at the costotransverse joint. During thoracic spine flexion and exhalation, the ribs typically glide superiorly and rotate anteriorly (figure 5.4).

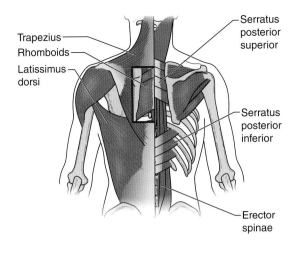

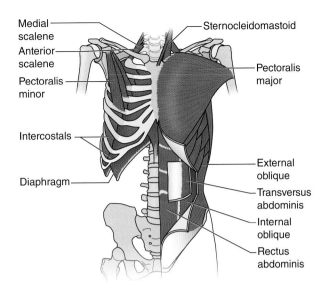

Posterior

Anterior

Figure 5.3 Muscles of the trunk.

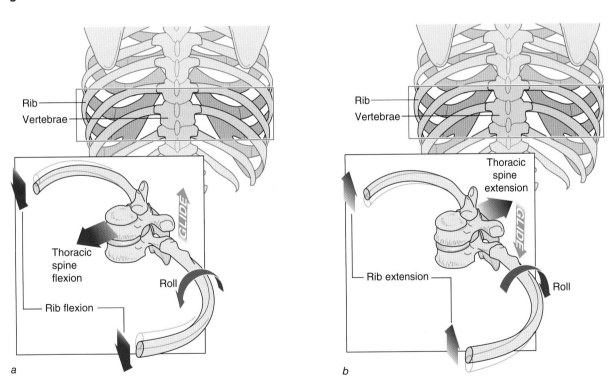

Figure 5.4 (a) Flexion and (b) extension of the thoracic spine and corresponding rib movement.

THORACIC SPINE JOINT ARTHROLOGY

Articular surfaces	Closed packed position	Resting position	Capsular pattern	ROM norms	End-feel
Cranial facet: concave Caudal facet: convex The facet joints are largely planar	Full extension	Midway between flexion and extension	Sidebending and rotation equally limited, extension	Flexion: 20–45° Extension: 25–45° Sidebending: 20–40° unilaterally Rotation: 35–50° unilaterally	Tissue stretch in all directions

Central Posterior-Anterior Nonthrust

Client position: Prone with head and spine in neutral.

Clinician position: Standing at client's head or to client's side if mobilizing lower segments.

Stabilization: Client's body serves as stabilization.

Mobilization: Multiple hand positions can be used for this technique, including thumb-over-thumb contact with the spinous process, bilateral ulnar borders lateral to the spinous processes, or the ulnar border of a single hand over the spinous process. The targeted segment is mobilized anteriorly toward the treatment table.

Goal of technique: To increase general thoracic spine motion.

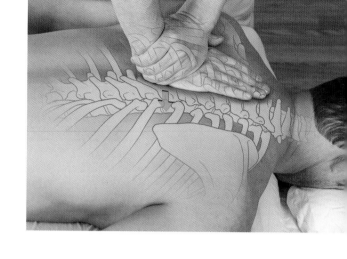

Note: Maintaining the elbows of the mobilizing arms in extension will reduce fatigue and promote mechanical advantage.

Unilateral Posterior-Anterior Nonthrust

Client position: Prone with head and spine neutral.

Clinician position: Standing at client's head or to client's side if mobilizing lower segments.

Stabilization: Client's body serves as stabilization.

Mobilization: Multiple hand positions can be used for this technique, including thumb-over-thumb contact with the transverse process, or the ulnar border of a single hand over the transverse process. The targeted segment is mobilized anteriorly toward the treatment table.

Goal of technique: To increase general thoracic spine motion.

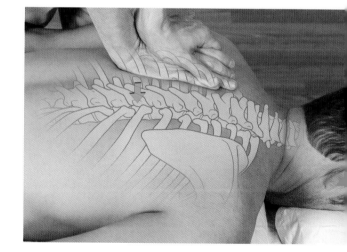

Notes: Maintaining the elbows of the mobilizing arms in extension will reduce fatigue and encourage mechanical advantage. If the superior or inferior segment is mobilized similarly on the contralateral side during this technique, joint gapping may increase.

Clinical tip: To determine thoracic spine positional faults, palpate the transverse processes of the client in prone position or sitting for symmetry in the cardinal planes. Then have the client move to prone on elbows before palpating again to confirm potential findings. This activity allows clinician to determine if a segment is positioned down and back or up and forward relative to adjacent segments.

Upper Thoracic Thrust

Client position: Supine with hands clasped around neck, elbows in front of body.

Clinician position: Standing to client's side with client's elbows stabilized in clinician's chest, and clinician's caudal forearm underneath client.

Stabilization: The client's elbows are held together near the chest.

Mobilization: The clinician's lower hand should make a fist with the distal interphalangeal joints extended, and place the target spinous processes between the fingertips and palm eminences. The clinician rolls the client onto this lower hand and performs a thrust in an anterior to posterior direction.

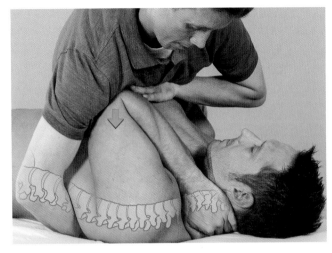

Goal of technique: To increase upper thoracic extension, general thoracic motion, and potentially, shoulder motion.

Notes: Various hand positions can be used, including the "pistol grip." Attempting to pull the thoracic segments caudally may help orient the facet joints closer to the horizontal plane prior to thrusting.

Clinical tip: Prior to performing high-velocity thrusts, ensure thorough subjective and objective exams have been performed to rule out red flag conditions, and exercise caution as needed. Also, for thrusts requiring a clinician to make a type of fist or grip, exercise caution to protect the phalanges as pressure is applied. A lip balm tube or other cylindrical item can be used in the palm to prevent injury to the clinician's hand.

Mid-Thoracic Bilateral Thrust

> *VIDEO 5.1* **in the web study guide shows this technique.**

Client position: Supine with arms across chest, hugging thorax tightly. Arm nearest clinician is below contralateral arm.

Clinician position: Standing to client's side, leaning on anterior surface of client's arms.

Stabilization: The clinician can use upper hand to keep client's arms wrapped tightly and positioned close to the upper trunk.

Mobilization: The clinician's lower hand should make a fist with the distal interphalangeal joints extended, and place the target spinous processes between fingertips and palm eminences. Clinician rolls client onto the lower hand and performs a thrust in an anterior to posterior direction.

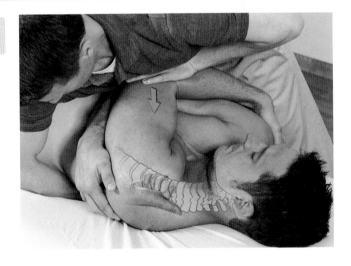

Goal of technique: To increase mid-thoracic extension and general thoracic motion.

Notes: Various hand positions can be used, including the "pistol grip." The clinician should flex the client's trunk until the client's trunk weight rests over the clinician's hand on the target segments.

Mid-Thoracic Unilateral Thrust

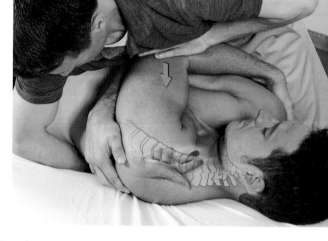

Client position: Supine with arms across chest, hugging thorax tightly. Arm nearest clinician should be below contralateral arm.

Clinician position: Standing to client's side, leaning on anterior surface of client's arms.

Stabilization: The clinician can use upper hand to keep client's arms wrapped tightly and positioned close to the upper trunk.

Mobilization: Clinician's lower hand should make a "pistol grip" with middle finger over the transverse process of the involved vertebra, and the thenar eminence over the contralateral transverse process of the vertebra below. The clinician rolls client onto the lower hand wrapped around the client and performs a thrust in an anterior to posterior direction.

Goal of technique: To increase mid-thoracic extension and general thoracic motion.

Note: The clinician should flex the client's trunk using crossed arms until the client's trunk weight rests over the clinician's hand on the target segments.

Mid-Thoracic Prone Rotator Thrust

 VIDEO 5.2 in the web study guide shows this technique.

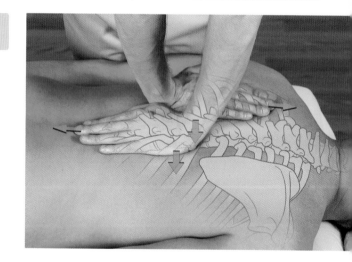

Client position: Prone with arms at sides to limit tension on thoracic musculature and other soft tissue.

Clinician position: Standing to client's side.

Stabilization: Clinician's cranial hand is placed over targeted segment's transverse process farthest from the clinician, with fingers pointed caudally. Clinician's caudal hand is placed over the targeted segment's nearest transverse process, with fingers pointed cranially. Preloading the overlying tissue by taking up its slack aids stabilization.

Mobilization: Clinician's caudal hand thrusts in a cranial and anterior direction, while cranial hand thrusts in a caudal and anterior direction.

Goal of technique: To increase mid-thoracic extension, general thoracic motion, and potentially, shoulder motion.

Note: Lowering the client below the waist level of the clinician will facilitate mechanical advantage and appropriate force application.

Thoracic Rotation Glide

Client position: Prone with head and spine neutral.

Clinician position: Standing to client's side.

Stabilization: Stabilization may or may not be needed; however, a stabilizing hand can hook over the spinous process of the segment inferior or superior to the one being mobilized.

Mobilization: Place 1 or both thumbs on the lateral surface of the spinous process of the segment to be mobilized; mobilize in a lateral direction.

Goal of technique: To increase thoracic spine rotation.

Note: The fingers of both hands can be used to stabilize the inferior and superior segments while using both thumbs to mobilize the target segment.

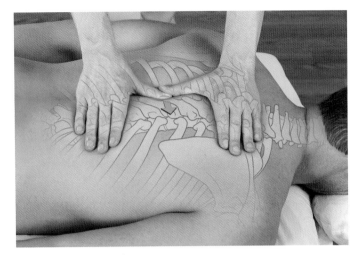

Thoracic Flexion Glide

Client position: Seated with hands clasped behind neck, elbows forward (or arms crossed in front of chest if there are shoulder motion limitations).

Clinician position: Standing at client's side, using 1 knee and thigh to support client's low back.

Stabilization: Using the thenar eminence, stabilizing hand is placed on superior portion of the spinous process of the segment inferior to the one being mobilized.

Mobilization: Mobilizing hand assists client into a flexion posture using client's elbows.

Goal of technique: To increase thoracic spine flexion.

Notes: The stabilizing hand will likely experience the most force during this mobilization and should remain firm on the inferior segment, as this technique is an indirect mobilization. Ensure the client is taken into sufficient flexion range of motion to produce movement at the target segment.

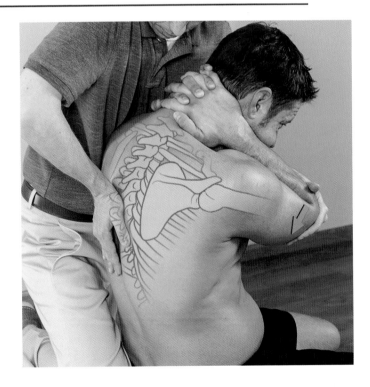

Thoracic Extension Glide

VIDEO 5.3 in the web study guide shows this technique.

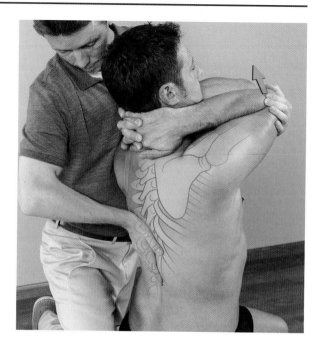

Client position: Seated with hands clasped behind neck, elbows forward (or arms crossed in front of chest if there are shoulder motion limitations).

Clinician position: Standing at client's side, using 1 knee and thigh to support client's low back.

Stabilization: Using the thenar eminence, stabilizing hand is placed on inferior portion of the spinous process of the segment inferior to the one being mobilized.

Mobilization: Mobilizing hand assists client into an extension posture using client's elbows.

Goal of technique: To increase thoracic spine extension.

Notes: The stabilizing hand will likely experience the most force during this mobilization and should remain firm on the inferior segment, as this technique is an indirect mobilization. Ensure the client is taken into sufficient extension range of motion to produce movement at the targeted segment.

Costotransverse Nonthrust

VIDEO 5.4 in the web study guide shows this technique.

Client position: Prone with arms relaxed at sides.

Clinician position: Standing at head of treatment table facing client (or to the side if lower segments are being mobilized).

Stabilization: Stabilizing hand maintains contact on the contralateral lamina and transverse process of the segment to be mobilized.

Mobilization: Mobilizing hand's thenar or hypothenar eminence mobilizes the most proximal portion of the rib in an anterior and slightly inferior direction.

Goal of technique: To facilitate movement of a hypomobile costovertebral joint.

Note: Maintaining the elbows of both arms in extension will reduce fatigue and promote mechanical advantage.

Seated First Rib Nonthrust Glide

Client position: Seated with head sidebent to the side of the rib being mobilized, putting slack on the ipsilateral scalene muscles. The contralateral arm is draped over the clinician's raised knee to put slack on the contralateral tissues and aid trunk support.

Clinician position: Standing behind client with metacarpophalangeal joint of index finger on medial aspect of the first rib. The contralateral knee is raised to provide a support for the client's contralateral upper extremity.

Stabilization: Clinician's stabilizing hand helps stabilize client's head in its sidebending position.

Mobilization: Mobilizing hand glides the medial aspect of the first rib in an inferior and medial direction. One suggested technique is to hold the rib still upon client inhalation, and then mobilize during exhalation.

Goal of technique: To depress an elevated first rib.

Note: The client's ipsilateral upper extremity can be rested on a bolster or the clinician's knee to provide more soft tissue slack.

Clinical tip: The Cervical Rotation Lateral Flexion Test (CRLF Test) allows a clinician to evaluate the presence of an elevated first rib. For this test, the seated client is moved passively into full cervical rotation to either direction, followed by full sidebending to the contralateral direction while maintaining the initial rotation. Limited sidebending compared to the uninvolved side indicates an elevated first rib on the same side as the limited sidebending.

Supine First Rib Nonthrust Glide

Client position: Supine with arms resting at sides.

Clinician position: Standing at head of treatment table facing client, cupping occiput with 1 hand; the metacarpophalangeal joint of the index finger (or web space) is on the medial aspect of the first rib to be treated.

Stabilization: The hand cupping the occiput stabilizes the head, maintaining it in a comfortable degree of sidebending to slacken the ipsilateral scalene muscles.

Mobilization: The mobilizing hand glides the first rib in an inferior and medial direction. One suggested technique is to hold the rib still upon client inhalation, and then mobilize during exhalation.

Goal of technique: To depress an elevated first rib.

Note: A similar technique can be performed with the client prone if the supine position is not possible.

Upper Rib Nonthrust

Client position: Supine with the involved side's upper extremity raised.

Clinician position: Standing near client's head on the involved side, holding client's arm with cranial hand proximal to elbow.

Stabilization: Clinician's caudal hand stabilizes the inferior rib using the thenar eminence or web space.

Mobilization: Clinician pulls client's raised upper extremity in a cranial direction, indirectly mobilizing the superior rib on the stabilized inferior rib.

Goal of technique: To correct either an exhalation restriction of the inferior rib or an inhalation restriction of the superior rib.

Note: In clients with shoulder motion limitations or pathology, direct mobilization through the ribs may be most appropriate.

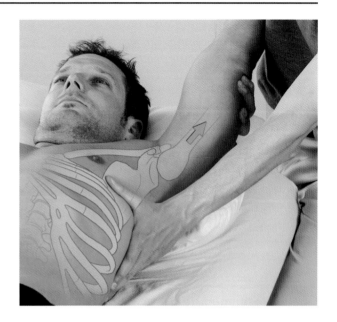

Lower Rib Nonthrust

Client position: Side-lying with the involved side nearest to ceiling.

Clinician position: Standing behind client, near head, holding client's arm with cranial hand proximal to elbow.

Stabilization: Clinician's caudal hand stabilizes the inferior rib using the thenar eminence or web space.

Mobilization: Clinician pulls client's raised upper extremity in a cranial direction, indirectly mobilizing the superior rib on the stabilized inferior rib.

Goal of technique: To correct either an exhalation restriction of the inferior rib or an inhalation restriction of the superior rib.

Note: In clients with shoulder motion limitations or pathology, direct mobilization through the ribs might be most appropriate.

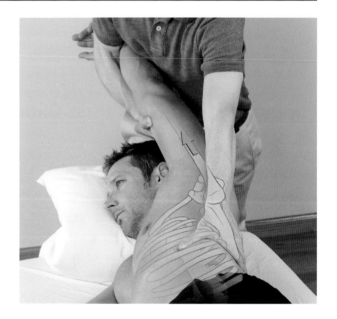

Go to the web study guide and complete the case study for this chapter. The case study discusses a 30-year-old male who reports mid-back pain after hiking in the mountains.

EVIDENCE FOR MANUAL THERAPY OF VARIOUS THORACIC SPINE AND REGIONAL JOINT PATHOLOGIES

Study	Clients	Intervention and comparison (if any)	Outcome(s)
Utilization of thrust and nonthrust mobilization for shoulder pain: Grade B			
Walser et al., 2009 (Level 1a)	3 studies (423 participants)	Usual medical care from general practitioners vs. MT + usual medical care MT vs. instructions for therapeutic exercise MT vs. other forms of physical therapy	MT group favored for shoulder pain and disability. MT favored for self-reported worst pain at 12-month follow-up. MT favored for shoulder complaints. Overall recommendation from study: MT for shoulder conditions may accelerate improvement, at least in the short term.
Strunce et al., 2009 (Level 2b)	21 participants	Thoracic spine and rib thrust	Immediate reduction in shoulder pain, increase in shoulder range of motion, and increase in patient-perceived global rating of change.
Utilization of thrust and nonthrust mobilization for neck pain: Grade B			
Walser et al., 2009 (Level 1a)	4 studies (186 participants)	Thoracic spine thrust (no comparison) Thoracic spine thrust vs. nonthrust MT Electrotherapy + massage vs. thoracic spine thrust + electrotherapy + massage Electro/thermal therapy vs. electro/thermal therapy + thoracic spine thrust	Immediate analgesic effects in patients with mechanical neck pain. Thoracic spine thrust results in greater short-term reductions in pain and disability than nonthrust MT. Inclusion of thoracic spine thrust results in greater reduction in neck pain and disability, and increases in cervical motion. Thoracic spine thrust results in greater reductions in pain and disability. Overall recommendation from study: there is sufficient evidence for use of thoracic spine manipulation for short-term results.
Martinez-Segura et al., 2012 (Level 1b)	90 participants	Cervical thrust vs. thoracic thrust	Similar reductions in pressure pain thresholds, neck pain intensity, and cervical spine range of motion.
Utilization of thrust and nonthrust mobilization for thoracic kyphosis: Grade D			
Bautmans et al., 2012 (Level 1b)	48 women (average age 76 years)	Thoracic nonthrust + taping + exercise vs. wait-list control	Intervention resulted in improved thoracic kyphosis compared to controls without serious adverse effects.

MT = manual therapy

6

LUMBAR SPINE AND PELVIS

LEARNING OBJECTIVES

After completing this chapter, you will be able to do the following:

◆ Describe the joint kinematics of the lumbar spine

◆ Demonstrate appropriate positioning, movements, and intentions for lumbar spine joint mobilization techniques

◆ Identify evidence supporting lumbar spine joint mobilization techniques

The lumbar spine is an intricate collection of joints surrounded by a dense fabric of soft tissues. Its function, either dynamically or statically, is crucial for nearly all functional activities. Some activities require smooth sliding of the lumbar spine's facet joints and coordinated motion of the vertebral segments on the intervertebral discs. For other activities, the lumbar spine must function as a stable support for the surrounding extremities, absorbing shock and serving as a base for muscle activity as necessary.

The function of the pelvis is no less important. Its shape is primed to attenuate forces. Its bones are thick, wide, and tall, and its articulations are strong to be efficient conduits of forces between the lower extremities and upper body. The architecture of the pelvic joints changes considerably over the lifespan, including during and after pregnancy. The importance of these joints necessitates clinicians have a sound understanding of how to treat dysfunctions using manual therapy techniques.

Anatomy

The lumbar spine is composed of 5 vertebrae and 5 pairs of facet joints (also called zygapophyseal joints). These vertebrae bear the most weight of any vertebrae in the spine, and the increased height of their vertebral bodies reflects this function. Vertebral discs exist between each lumbar segment and aid in shock absorption and facilitation of lumbar motion. The transverse processes of the lumbar spine are generally parallel to the spinous processes (figure 6.1).

The diarthrodial facet joints of the lumbar spine are formed by a capsule surrounding the superior and inferior articular processes of adjacent vertebrae. The orientation of these planar facet joints largely facilitates sagittal plane movements of flexion and extension. The superior articular processes face medially and slightly posteriorly, while the inferior articular processes face laterally and slightly anteriorly.

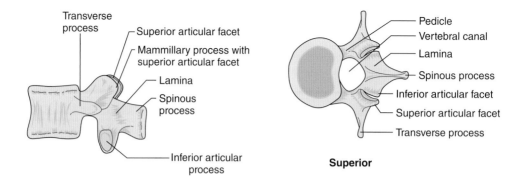

Figure 6.1 Lumbar spine facet joints.

The soft tissues surrounding the lumbar spine are unique. The supporting ligaments are thicker and stronger in the lumbar spine than the thoracic and cervical spines given the comparative loads it must bear. These ligaments include, from anterior to posterior, the anterior longitudinal ligament, posterior longitudinal ligament, intertransverse ligaments, ligamentum flavum, interspinous liga-

ment, and supraspinous ligament. The surrounding muscles range greatly in size from the segmental multifidi to the broad latissimus dorsi and thick erector spinae (figure 6.2).

Below the lumbar spine structures sit the sacroiliac joints. The sacroiliac joint on the posterior portion of the pelvis is composed of a convex iliac surface and the concave auricular surface of the sacrum,

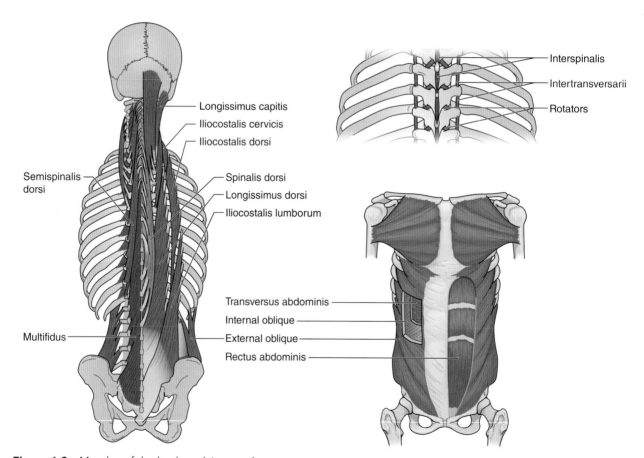

Figure 6.2 Muscles of the lumbopelvic complex.

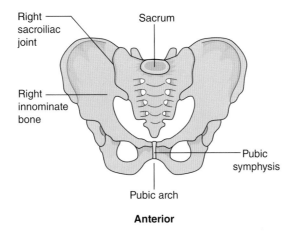

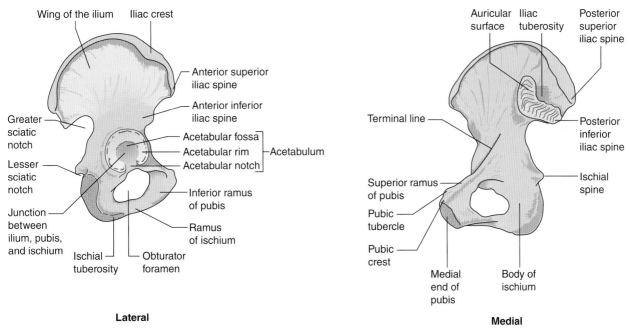

Figure 6.3 Aspects of the pelvis.

surrounded by a synovial capsule (figure 6.3). The bony congruity of these surfaces varies largely depending on the age of the client. In children, the surfaces are likely to be smooth and planar. With age, however, the surfaces develop ridges to provide joint support and aid force transfer. In the elderly client, the sacroiliac joint may be fused. On the anterior portion of the pelvis, the pubic symphysis is a fibrocartilaginous joint composed of the two pubic bones, separated by an interpubic disc. This joint has limited movement, and its surfaces can be considered mostly planar.

Similar to the lumbar spine, the sacroiliac joints are surrounded by dense soft tissues. A web of ligamentous connections serves to stabilize these largely planar joints, including the anterior sacroiliac ligaments, interosseous sacroiliac ligaments, sacrotuberous ligaments, and dorsal sacroiliac ligaments (figure 6.4). Interestingly, no muscles act directly to influence movement of the sacroiliac joints; however, many muscles influence the joints' motion. Such muscles include the gluteals, abdominals, hamstrings, adductors, and hip flexors.

Joint Kinematics

To describe the joint kinematics of the lumbar spine, the motion of the superior vertebrae's articular processes on the inferior vertebrae's articular processes will be detailed (e.g., L3 on L4). During

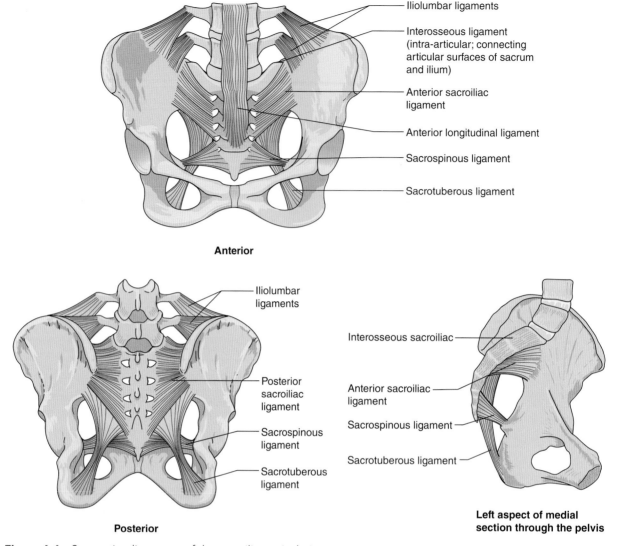

Anterior

Posterior

**Left aspect of medial
section through the pelvis**

Figure 6.4 Supporting ligaments of the sacroiliac articulations.

lumbar spine flexion, the inferior articular facets of the superior vertebrae (e.g., L3) move superiorly and anteriorly (up and forward) on the superior articular facets of the inferior vertebrae (e.g., L4). Lumbar spine extension involves opposite motions, as the uppermost facets glide inferiorly and posteriorly (down and back) on the lowermost facets (figure 6.5). Right rotation of a superior vertebrae on its inferior counterpart will create gapping of the ipsilateral facet joint on the right and close the contralateral facet on the left. Right lumbar spine side bending is a result of the ipsilateral (right) articular processes gliding inferiorly while the contralateral (left) articular processes glide superiorly (figure 6.6).

Innominate and sacroiliac kinematics occur in multiple planes (figure 6.7). Bilateral pelvic

motion, either anterior or posterior pelvic rotation, often accompanies motion at the lumbar spine or hips. For example, end-range hip flexion often accompanies posterior pelvic rotation, and posterior pelvic rotation often accompanies lumbar spine extension. Conversely, end-range hip extension often accompanies anterior pelvic rotation, and anterior pelvic rotation often accompanies lumbar spine flexion. End-range hip abduction and adduction are associated with ipsilateral innominate elevation and depression, respectively. Similarly, end-range hip external and internal rotation are associated with ipsilateral outflaring (lateral rotation) and inflaring (medial rotation) of the innominate, respectively.

An innominate may move independent of its other half, causing one of the following

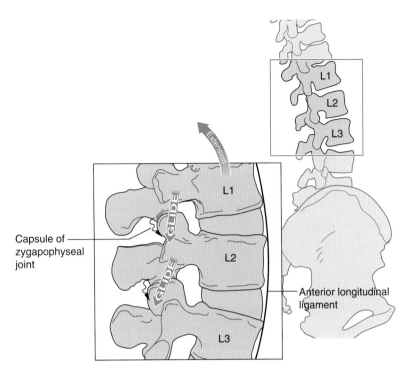

Figure 6.5 Lumbar spine facet motion during extension.

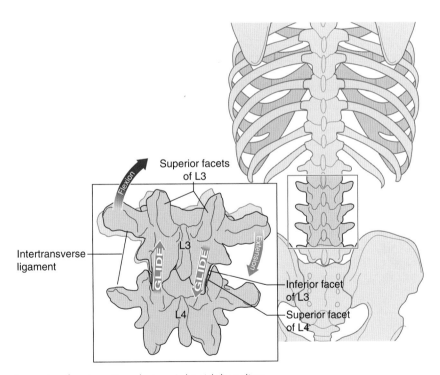

Figure 6.6 Lumbar spine facet motion during right sidebending.

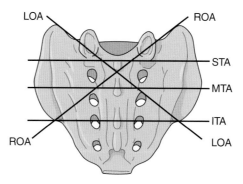

Figure 6.7 Commonly described axes of motion about the sacroiliac joint. LOA = left oblique axis; ROA = right oblique axis; STA = superior transverse axis; MTA = middle transverse axis; ITA = inferior transverse axis.

dysfunctions: (1) posteriorly rotated innominate; (2) anteriorly rotated innominate; (3) inflared innominate (when the ASIS moves medially); (4) outflared innominate (when the ASIS moves laterally); (5) upslip (when the entire innominate moves superiorly); or (6) downslip (when the entire innominate moves inferiorly).

The joint kinematics of the sacroiliac joint include 5 primary motions. Nutation (flexion of the sacrum) and counternutation (extension of the sacrum) are the most commonly described motions (figure 6.8). Other motions described include anterior torsion (anterior motion of one sacral base), posterior torsion (posterior motion of one sacral base), and sidebending (inferior motion of one side of the sacrum and/or superior motion of the contralateral side). Although minimal movement occurs at the pubic symphysis, one pubic bone may move inferiorly or superiorly on the other.

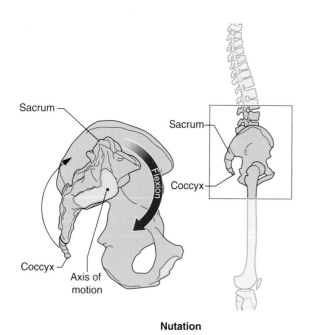

Nutation

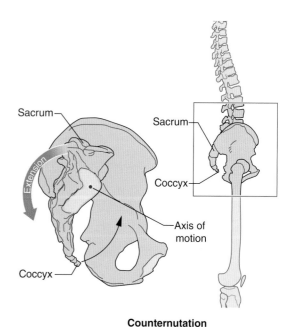

Counternutation

Figure 6.8 Joint kinematic motions of the sacrum.

LUMBAR SPINE AND SACROILIAC JOINT ARTHROLOGY

Articular surfaces	Closed packed position	Resting position	Capsular pattern	ROM norms	End-feel
Lumbar spine					
Cranial facet: concave Caudal facet: convex The facet joints are largely planar	Full extension	Midway between flexion and extension	Sidebending and rotation equally limited, extension	Flexion: 40–60° Extension: 20–35° Sidebending: 15–20° unilaterally Rotation: 3–18° unilaterally	Tissue stretch in all directions
Sacroiliac					
Sacrum: concave Ilia: convex	Nutation	Neutral	Pain when the joints are stressed	Minimal movement	Tissue stretch in all directions

Hook-Lying Nonthrust Distraction

Client position: Supine with bilateral hips and knees flexed with feet on treatment table (hook-lying).

Clinician position: Standing at foot of treatment table facing client.

Stabilization: No direct stabilization required.

Mobilization: Clinician places hands around proximal aspect of client's calves or distal thighs, and mobilization is imparted with a gradual leaning backward by clinician to produce distraction to lumbar spine.

Goal of technique: To increase general lumbar spine motion.

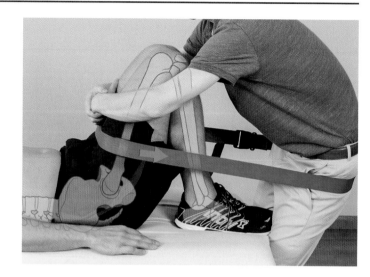

Notes: This technique may also be done with a belt around the proximal thighs. It can be an indicator of the beneficial use of mechanical traction.

Sitting Nonthrust Distraction

Client position: Sitting upright on treatment table with arms crossed across chest, sitting near back edge of table.

Clinician position: Standing directly behind client, clinician places a pillow between clinician and client and grasps client's most caudal elbow.

Stabilization: No direct stabilization required.

Mobilization: A distraction force is provided through caudal elbow in a cranial direction. The distraction force can be used with client's breathing pattern.

Goal of technique: To increase general lumbar spine motion.

Note: The line of distraction force may need to be slightly posterior depending on the angle of client's lean from vertical.

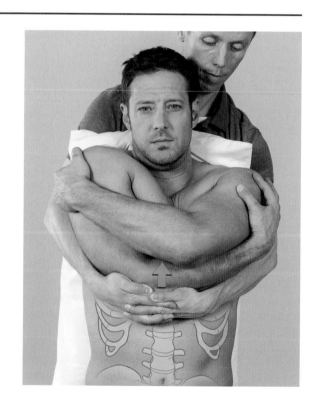

Side-Lying Nonthrust Distraction

Client position: Side-lying (with involved side up if unilateral distraction is performed), with hips flexed 60 to 90°. Clinician rotates spine down to cranial vertebra of segments to be treated.

Clinician position: Standing directly in front of client at level of dysfunction.

Stabilization: Cranial forearm and hand are placed against spine with index and middle fingers fixating cranial vertebra of segments to be treated.

Mobilization: Caudal arm and hand are placed on sacrum with index and middle fingers on caudal vertebra of segments to be treated. Clinician applies a traction force, moving caudal arm and body (which is contacting client's upper legs) as a unit in a caudal direction.

Goal of technique: To increase general lumbar spine motion.

Note: This distraction is useful when specific dysfunctional segments are identified.

Quadruped Flexion Glide

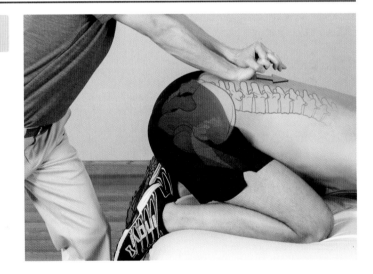

VIDEO 6.1 in the web study guide shows this technique.

Client position: Quadruped with hands and knees hip-width apart.

Clinician position: Standing behind client (or to either side if such positioning is necessary to reach segment to be treated).

Stabilization: No direct stabilization required.

Mobilization: Using firm contact of the pisiform or thumbs on spinous process of vertebra to be mobilized, client rocks buttocks toward heels while the clinician maintains a cranially directed force with mobilizing hand(s).

Goal of technique: To increase lumbar spine flexion.

Note: A low treatment table typically aids efficient clinician body mechanics.

Clinical tip: To determine lumbar spine positional faults, palpate the transverse processes of the client in prone for symmetry in all cardinal planes. Then have the client move into either quadruped or prone on elbows before palpating again to confirm potential findings. This activity allows a clinician to determine if a segment is positioned down and back or up and forward relative to adjacent segments.

Side-Lying Flexion Glide

Client position: Side-lying (with involved side up if a unilateral dysfunction exists), with hips and knees flexed 60 to 90°. Clinician rotates spine down to cranial vertebra of segment to be treated.

Clinician position: Standing directly in front of client at level of dysfunction.

Stabilization: Cranial hand fixates transverse process or spinous process of cranial vertebra of dysfunctional segment.

Mobilization: Caudal hand (placed on caudal vertebra) and body of clinician mobilize segment as a unit to produce flexion of spine.

Goal of technique: To increase lumbar spine flexion.

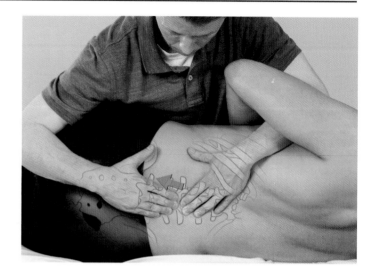

Note: This mobilization is used for flexion or "opening" of a lumbar spine segment, aiding in the correction of a "closing" restriction (when a facet is stuck down and back).

Side-Lying Extension Glide

 VIDEO 6.2 in the web study guide shows this technique.

Client position: Side-lying (with involved side up if a unilateral dysfunction exists). Clinician rotates spine down to cranial vertebra of segment to be treated.

Clinician position: Standing directly in front of client at level of dysfunction, clinician places client's knees in clinician's anterior hip region.

Stabilization: Index finger of cranial hand stabilizes spinous process of cranial vertebra of dysfunctional segment.

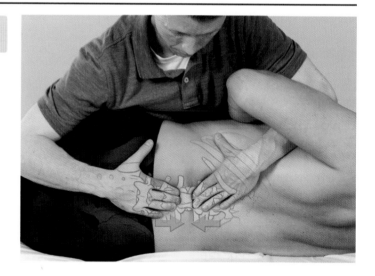

Mobilization: Caudal hand is placed over transverse processes of caudal vertebra. Extension mobilization is produced by moving client's lower extremities and pelvis in a dorsal direction and attempting to approximate spinous processes of desired segment.

Goal of technique: To increase lumbar spine extension.

Notes: Knee and hip joint angles remain fixed during mobilization. This mobilization attempts to extend or "close" the lumbar spine segment, correcting an "opening" restriction (when a facet is stuck up and forward).

Posterior-Anterior Nonthrust

Client position: Prone with legs extended and arms relaxed.

Clinician position: Standing at client's side.

Stabilization: No direct stabilization required.

Mobilization: The pisiform or thumbs are placed over spinous process of the level to be mobilized. Mobilizing hand glides vertebrae via spinous process ventrally. The other hand may be used to guide mobilizing hand or provide additional force.

Goal of technique: To increase general lumbar spine motion.

Note: This mobilization is also used to aid nutrition to articular surfaces by facilitating fluid diffusion around the lumbar discs.

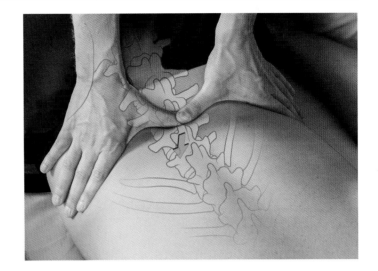

Cranial Glide Distraction

Client position: Prone with legs extended and arms relaxed. Lumbar spine is in a resting position or slightly flexed.

Clinician position: Standing at client's side.

Stabilization: Caudal hand is positioned with thumb on spinous process of the more caudal vertebra.

Mobilization: Cranial hand is positioned with thumb or pisiform over the most caudal surface of the spinous process of the cranial vertebra. Manipulating hand glides spinous process cranially and ventrally (up and forward).

Goal of technique: To increase lumbar spine flexion of the targeted segment.

Notes: This mobilization may also facilitate extension of the segment superior to the targeted segment as its spinous processes are approximated. The client may place a pillow under abdomen for comfort.

Cranial Glide Approximation

Client position: Prone with legs extended and arms relaxed. Lumbar spine is in a resting position or slightly flexed.

Clinician position: Standing at client's side.

Stabilization: Cranial hand is positioned with thumb on spinous process of the more cranial vertebra.

Mobilization: Caudal hand is positioned with thumb or pisiform over the most caudal surface of spinous process of caudal vertebra. Manipulating hand glides the spinous process cranially and ventrally (up and forward).

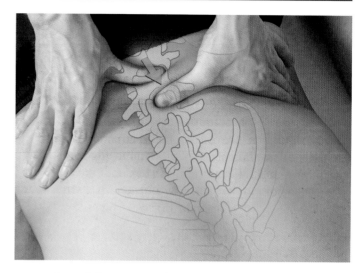

Goal of technique: To increase lumbar spine extension of the targeted segment.

Notes: This mobilization may also facilitate flexion of the segment inferior to the targeted segment as its spinous processes are distracted. The client may place a pillow under abdomen for comfort.

Prone Gapping Glide

Client position: Prone with legs extended and arms relaxed. Lumbar spine is in a resting position.

Clinician position: Standing at client's side at level of dysfunction.

Stabilization: Caudal hand is positioned with second and third fingers on lateral surface of spinous process of the more caudal vertebra, opposite the side to which the nearest facet joint will be gapped.

Mobilization: Cranial hand is positioned with thumb on lateral surface of spinous process of the more cranial vertebra on same side nearest facet joint will be

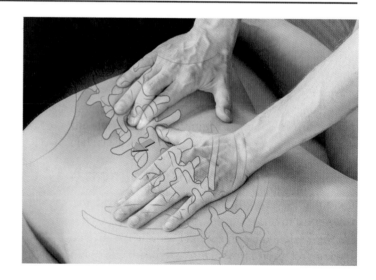

gapped. Cranial vertebra's spinous process is moved laterally, away from clinician, gapping the nearest facet joint.

Goal of technique: To help reduce a rotational positional fault; may also release impinged meniscoid tissue of facet joints or reduce a herniated disc.

Note: The client may place a pillow under abdomen for comfort.

Side-Lying Gapping Glide

Client position: Side-lying with top arm over clinician's mobilizing arm. Client's knees are moved toward clinician until movement is felt at target segment. Upper trunk is rotated away from clinician until motion is detected at target segment.

Clinician position: Standing in front of client.

Stabilization: Caudal hand is positioned with 2 fingers on lateral surface of the caudal vertebra's spinous process, opposite the side to which nearest facet joint will be gapped.

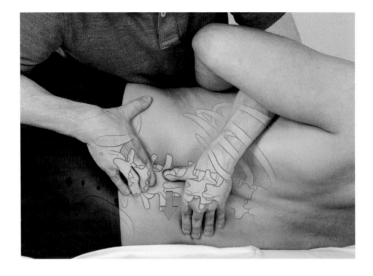

Mobilization: Cranial hand's thumb is positioned on lateral surface of spinous process of the more cranial vertebra on the same side the nearest facet joint will be gapped. Cranial vertebra's spinous process is moved laterally, away from clinician, gapping nearest facet joint.

Goal of technique: To help reduce a rotational positional fault; may also release impinged meniscoid tissue of the facet joints.

Note: The client may place a pillow under the side of the abdomen for comfort.

Prone Sidebending Glide

Client position: Prone with legs extended and arms relaxed. Lumbar spine is in a resting position.

Clinician position: Standing at client's side.

Stabilization: Cranial hand is positioned with thumb or index finger on far side of spinous process of the more cranial vertebra.

Mobilization: Caudal hand grasps medial surface of distal thigh nearest clinician, using arm to support client's lower leg. Cli-

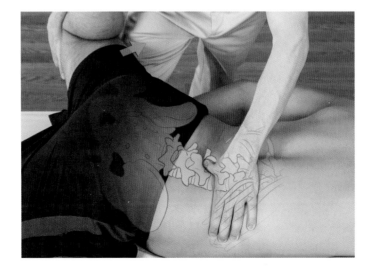

nician then moves the leg into abduction, through end range, imparting a sidebending force to the more caudal vertebra.

Goal of technique: To help reduce a sidebending positional fault and increase lumbar sidebending.

Note: The client may place a pillow under the abdomen for comfort.

Side-Lying Sidebending Glide ("Breaking the Bread")

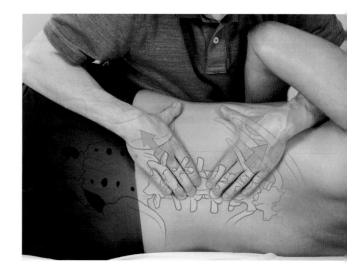

Client position: Side-lying with legs relaxed and top arm resting over clinician's cranial forearm.

Clinician position: Standing to client's front at level of dysfunction.

Stabilization: No direct stabilization required.

Mobilization: Clinician hooks fingers under spinous processes of segment(s) to be mobilized and pulls them laterally (toward ceiling) while forearms push thorax and pelvis away from each other. Clinician primarily uses his or her body-weight to glide iliac crest caudally.

Goal of technique: To help reduce a sidebending positional fault and increase lumbar sidebending.

Notes: This glide may be performed as a thrust/manipulation. The clinician may also grasp only the medial aspect of the client's nearest paraspinals to mobilize the paraspinal soft tissues in attempt to reduce muscle spasm.

Lumbar Gapping Thrust

 VIDEO 6.3 **in the web study guide shows this technique.**

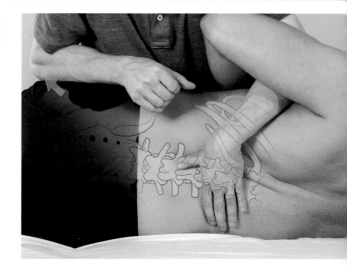

Client position: Side-lying with dysfunctional side up holding wrists. Bottom leg is extended; top hip is flexed until movement is felt at target segment; top foot rests behind bottom leg.

Clinician position: Standing to client's front with cranial arm through client's top arm. Clinician's caudal forearm is placed on the gluteal mass.

Stabilization: Clinician rotates thoracic spine until it is approximately 45° to table or until movement is felt at level of dysfunction. Clinician stabilizes spinous process of superior segment of the manipulation with cranial thumb.

Mobilization: Clinician thrusts anteriorly and inferiorly in relation to client's body with caudal forearm over the gluteal mass.

Goal of technique: To gap a closed lumbar facet joint.

Note: The angle of thrust may vary depending on the orientation of the client and the level of the dysfunctional lumbar segment.

Clinical tip: Prior to performing high-velocity thrusts, ensure thorough subjective and objective exams have been performed first to rule out red flag conditions, and exercise caution as needed. Red flag conditions include fractures, stress to surgical graft sites, rheumatoid arthritis, and osteoarthritis. Pregnancy and disc prolapse also warrant caution.

Lumbar Down-and-Back Thrust

Client position: Side-lying with dysfunctional side up, hands grasping opposite wrists. Bottom leg is extended; top hip is flexed until movement is felt at target segment; top foot rests behind bottom leg.

Clinician position: Standing to client's front with cranial arm through client's arms. Clinician's caudal forearm is placed on the gluteal mass.

Stabilization: Clinician rotates thoracic spine until movement is felt at target segment. Clinician stabilizes spinous process of superior segment with cranial thumb.

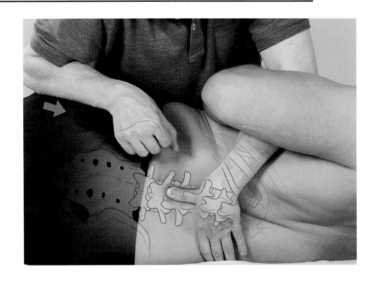

Mobilization: Clinician thrusts posteriorly and superiorly in relation to client's body with caudal forearm over the gluteal mass.

Goal of technique: To close a lumbar facet joint stuck in an open position (i.e., up and forward).

Notes: Rotating the client toward the body of the clinician may aid body mechanics and allow more compression. Thrust force may also be applied through the cranial thumb; however, only 20% of the thrust force is recommended to be imparted in this way. It should only be a minor force contributor.

Posterior Innominate Rotation

 VIDEO 6.4 **in the web study guide shows this technique.**

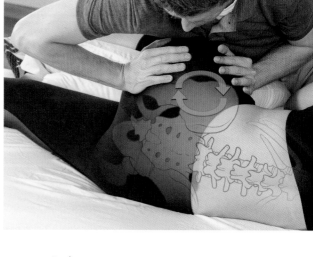

Client position: Side-lying with involved side up and hip and knee flexed to 90°; uninvolved hip and knee neutral.

Clinician position: Standing to front of client at level of hips.

Stabilization: Client's extended lower extremity nearest treatment table serves to stabilize the innominate.

Mobilization: Clinician places one hand on the superior iliac crest with palm over anterior superior iliac spine. Other hand is placed inferiorly over the ischial tuberosity. Both hands are used on the respective bony prominences to rotate the innominate posteriorly.

Goal of technique: To correct an anteriorly rotated innominate.

Note: It may be helpful for the clinician to lean over the client to gain mechanical advantage.

Anterior Innominate Rotation

 VIDEO 6.5 **in the web study guide shows this technique.**

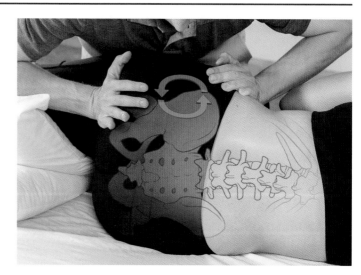

Client position: Side-lying with involved side up, with hip and knee 0° flexion, and uninvolved (lower) hip and knee flexed to 90°.

Clinician position: Standing at front of client at hip level.

Stabilization: Client's flexed uninvolved extremity nearest treatment table serves to stabilize the innominate.

Mobilization: Clinician places one hand on the superior iliac crest. Other hand is placed inferiorly over the ischial tuberosity. Both hands are used on the respective bony prominences to rotate the innominate anteriorly.

Goal of technique: To correct a posteriorly rotated innominate.

Note: It may be helpful for the clinician to lean over the client to gain mechanical advantage.

Prone Outflare Glide

Client position: Prone with arms not obstructing pelvis.

Clinician position: Standing or sitting next to innominate to be treated.

Stabilization: Client's body weight serves as stabilizing force.

Mobilization: Clinician places one hand lateral to posterior superior iliac spine on involved side. This hand provides a medial force to the posterior superior iliac spine during mobilization. Other hand grasps the ipsilateral anterior superior iliac spine and pulls it laterally.

Goal of technique: To correct an inflared innominate.

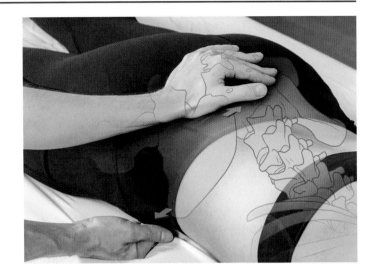

Notes: It may be helpful to squat or sit so the elbows of the clinician can be straightened and used in the frontal plane of the client. A pillow can be placed beneath the client's abdomen for comfort if needed.

Supine Outflare Glide

Client position: Supine with hip to be treated flexed to 90°.

Clinician position: Standing next to hip to be treated with flexed extremity's knee between his or her caudal hand and trunk.

Stabilization: Client's body weight serves as stabilizing force in addition to clinician's hand and trunk surrounding knee.

Mobilization: Clinician supinates cranial hand, places palm over anterior superior iliac spine, and mobilizes the innominate in a posterior-lateral direction.

Goal of technique: To correct an inflared innominate.

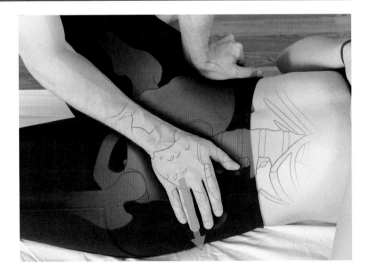

Note: Ensure that the elbow of the mobilizing hand is near extension and medial to the anterior superior iliac spine to mobilize in the correct direction using the weight of the body.

Inflare Glide

Client position: Supine with arms not obstructing pelvis.

Clinician position: Clinician stands or sits next to the innominate to be treated.

Stabilization: Client's body weight serves as stabilizing force.

Mobilization: Clinician places one hand lateral to anterior superior iliac spine on involved side. This hand provides a medial force to the anterior superior iliac spine during mobilization. Other hand grasps the ipsilateral posterior superior iliac spine and pulls it laterally.

Goal of technique: To correct an out-flared innominate.

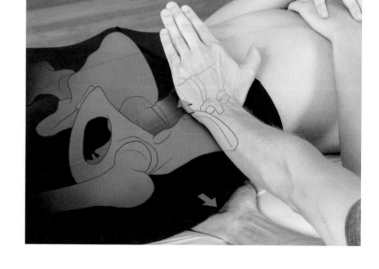

Note: It is helpful to squat or sit so the elbows of the clinician can be straightened and used in the frontal plane of the client.

Inferior Innominate Glide

Client position: Prone with lower legs near end of treatment table.

Clinician position: Standing at client's feet, facing client.

Stabilization: Client's body weight serves as stabilizing force.

Mobilization: Clinician grasps affected lower extremity around ankle with both hands and lifts it into available range of hip extension and provides an inferiorly directed force.

Goal of technique: To correct an innominate upslip dysfunction.

Note: The client may grasp the treatment table if further stabilization is needed.

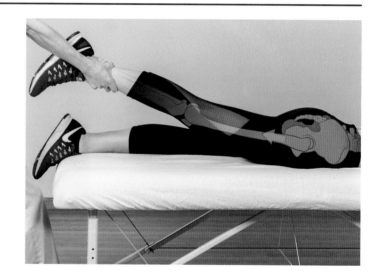

Superior Innominate Glide

Client position: Prone with lower extremity and innominate of side to be treated off edge of treatment table. Client's toe may rest on ground, or ankle may be braced between clinician's thighs. Client's leg can also be placed on a stool.

Clinician position: Standing at client's side, facing client's head.

Stabilization: Client's body weight serves as stabilizing force.

Mobilization: Clinician places heel of one hand on inferior surface of ischial tuberosity and mobilizes it in a superior/cephalic direction.

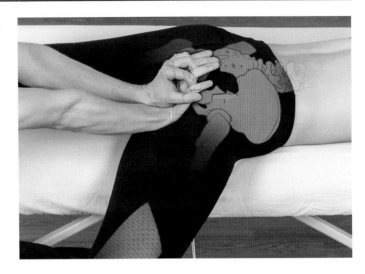

Goal of technique: To correct an innominate downslip dysfunction.

Notes: The client may grasp the edge of the treatment table if needed. The clinician can adjust the degree of hip flexion to adjust the position of the innominate as needed. The elbow of the mobilizing arm should be extended for mechanical advantage.

Inferior Pubic Glide

Client position: Supine.

Clinician position: Standing toward head of treatment table facing client's feet.

Stabilization: Client's body weight serves as stabilizing force.

Mobilization: Clinician places one hand on top of the other with heel of bottom hand just lateral to the pubic symphysis on the superior aspect of the pubic ramus. Clinician mobilizes the pubis in an inferior direction.

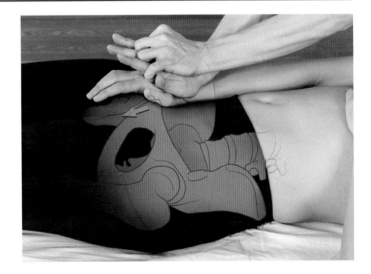

Goal of technique: To correct a superior fault of a pubic bone.

Notes: The clinician should ensure that his or her fingers are extended for the comfort of the client. The clinician can have the client locate the pubic bones independently and mobilize over his or her hand for increased comfort.

Superior Pubic Glide

Client position: Supine.

Clinician position: Standing toward foot of treatment table facing client's head.

Stabilization: Client's body weight serves as stabilizing force.

Mobilization: Clinician places one hand on top of the other with heel of bottom hand just lateral to the pubic symphysis on the inferior aspect of the pubic ramus. Clinician mobilizes the pubis in a superior direction.

Goal of technique: To correct an inferior fault of a pubic bone.

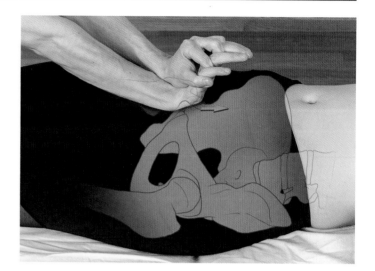

Notes: The clinician should ensure that his or her fingers are extended for the comfort of the client. The clinician can have the client locate the pubic bones independently and mobilize over his or her hand for increased comfort.

Bilateral Sacral Sidebending Glide

Client position: Prone with a pillow beneath abdomen to limit lumbar spine lordosis.

Clinician position: Standing to side of client at level of sacroiliac joints.

Stabilization: Ulnar aspect of clinician's cranial hand is placed on contralateral sacral base to provide a stabilizing force in an inferior direction.

Mobilization: Ulnar aspect of caudal hand is placed on inferior aspect of ipsilateral inferior lateral angle. The clinician mobilizes the ipsilateral side of the sacrum in a superior direction.

Goal of technique: To correct a sidebent sacrum.

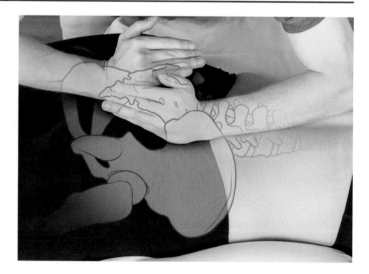

Note: To optimize the mechanical advantage and direction of mobilization, the clinician's forearms should be near the horizontal plane of the sacrum.

Unilateral Sacral Sidebending Glide

Client position: Prone with a pillow beneath abdomen to limit lumbar spine lordosis.

Clinician position: Standing inferior to sacroiliac joint.

Stabilization: Client's body weight serves as stabilizing force.

Mobilization: Clinician places one hand on top of other with heel of bottom hand on inferior aspect of ipsilateral inferior lateral angle. Clinician mobilizes ipsilateral side of sacrum in a superior direction.

Goal of technique: To correct a sidebent sacrum.

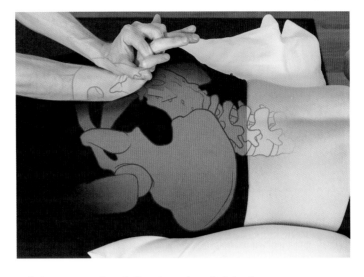

Note: To optimize the mechanical advantage and direction of mobilization, the clinician's forearms should be near the horizontal plane of the sacrum.

Sacral Rotation for a Posteriorly Sheared Sacrum

Client position: Prone with a pillow beneath abdomen to limit lumbar spine lordosis.

Clinician position: Standing to side of client, opposite side to be treated.

Stabilization: Client's body against treatment table serves as stabilizing force.

Mobilization: Clinician places one hand on top of the other with heel of bottom hand on the sacral base of the side to be treated. Clinician mobilizes the sacral base in an anterior direction.

Goal of technique: To correct a posteriorly sheared pelvic base.

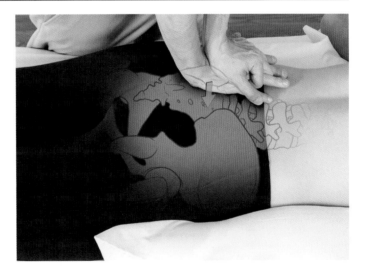

Note: Positioning the client near the edge of the table may facilitate the clinician's mechanical advantage.

Sacral Rotation for an Anteriorly Sheared Sacrum

Client position: Prone with a pillow beneath abdomen to limit lumbar spine lordosis.

Clinician position: Clinician stands to side of client at level of sacroiliac joint.

Stabilization: Stabilizing hand is placed over nearest posterior superior iliac spine to prevent posterior displacement of the innominate. Client's body against treatment table will also serve as stabilization.

Mobilization: Clinician places mobilizing hand over inferior lateral angle farthest from the clinician and provides an anteriorly directed force.

Goal of technique: To correct an anteriorly sheared sacral base contralateral to the inferior lateral angle being mobilized.

Note: Positioning the client near the edge of the table may facilitate the clinician's mechanical advantage.

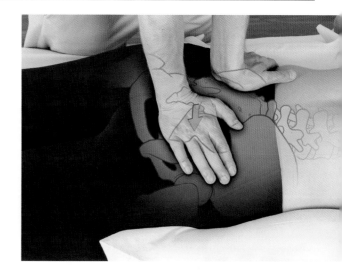

Supine Sacroiliac Thrust

 VIDEO 6.6 in the web study guide shows this technique.

Client position: Client is supine with fingers interlaced behind neck, elbows together under chin. Pelvis is placed on side of treatment table nearest clinician; feet and head are positioned toward opposite side. Ankles are crossed.

Clinician position: Clinician places cranial arm through spaces between client's forearms and upper arms, rotates client's body toward clinician, and fixes cranial hand on treatment table.

Stabilization: Stabilizing hand is cranial hand placed on table with clinician's body weight. Client should be rolled only until contralateral ilium lifts from table.

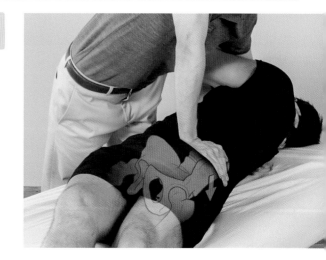

Mobilization: Clinician places mobilizing hand over the contralateral anterior superior iliac spine and thrusts posteriorly.

Goal of technique: This thrust is a nonspecific technique for the sacroiliac joint.

Note: The clinician should ensure the client maintains contralateral trunk sidebending after rolling.

Clinical tips: Clinicians and clients should understand that a "pop" is not necessary, and it may not relate to clinical outcomes. Thrust techniques may be attempted twice in the absence of a "pop" or cavitation.

Side-Lying Sacroiliac Thrust

VIDEO 6.7 **in the web study guide shows this technique.**

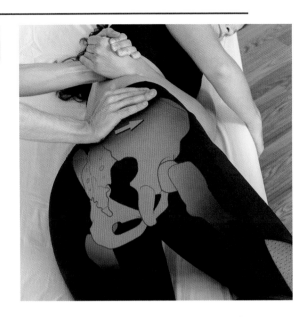

Client position: Side-lying with dysfunctional side up. Bottom leg is extended, and top hip is flexed until top foot is able to rest behind bottom leg. Uppermost knee rests slightly off treatment table. Uppermost hand grasps table. Lowermost hand reaches backward by waist to grasp clinician's hand, maintaining elbow contact with table.

Clinician position: Standing behind client with cranial hand grasping client's hand. Clinician's caudal hand is cupped around the uppermost posterior superior iliac spine.

Stabilization: Client aids stabilization by maintaining contact with lowermost elbow and table.

Mobilization: Clinician thrusts through caudal hand around posterior superior iliac spine in an anterior and lateral direction relative to client.

Goal of technique: This thrust is a nonspecific technique for the sacroiliac joint.

Note: To optimize thrust mechanics, the clinician should place his or her caudal lower extremity in extension and his or her cranial lower extremity in a flexed, lunge position.

Go to the web study guide and complete the case study for this chapter. The case study discusses a 25-year-old female indoor soccer player.

EVIDENCE FOR MANUAL THERAPY OF VARIOUS LUMBAR SPINE AND PELVIS JOINT PATHOLOGIES

Study	Clients	Intervention and comparison (if any)	Outcome(s)
Utilization of thrust and nonthrust mobilization for lumbar radiculopathy: Grade B			
Leininger et al., 2011 (Level 1a)	11 studies (2,132 participants)	MT vs. traction, exercise, or corset use MT vs. heat MT vs. chemonucleolysis MT vs. sham MT MT vs. medication, massage and diathermy, bed rest, back school, or placebo ointment MT vs modalities, stabilization exercise, or no treatment MT + exercise vs. exercise or control MT vs. exercise MT + home exercise vs. exercise or education MT + exercise + hydrotherapy vs. bed rest or education MT vs. traction	MT favored over other conditions for pain and subjective improvement. MT favored for pain. MT favored for pain and disability. MT favored for pain. MT favored for pain, disability, finger-floor distance, and straight leg raise. MT favored for disability. Stabilization exercise favored for pain, dysfunction, and disability; both MT and stabilization exercise favored over control. MT favored for pain. Exercise favored for pain; MT + home exercise and exercise favored over education. MT + exercise + hydrotherapy favored for pain and disability. MT favored for pain. Overall recommendation from study: moderate evidence that MT is effective for acute symptoms; low quality evidence supports MT for chronic symptoms.
Utilization of thrust and nonthrust mobilization for low back pain: Grade B			
Bronfort et al., 2004 (Level 1a)	31 studies (5,202 participants)	Various grouping of MT +/- exercise vs. PT, general practice medical care, NSAIDs, diathermy, exercise, education, soft tissue therapy or control	Moderate evidence that MT has better short-term efficacy for acute LBP than diathermy. Limited evidence that MT has better short-term efficacy for acute LBP than diathermy + exercise + education. Moderate evidence that MT + exercise is similar in effect for CLBP to NSAIDs + exercise in the short and long term. Moderate evidence that MT is superior for CLBP to PT and home exercise for reducing long-term disability. Moderate evidence that MT is superior for CLBP to general practice medical care and placebo in the short term and superior to PT in the long term for patient improvement. Moderate evidence that MT is superior to education for pain reduction for mixed acute and chronic LBP in the short term. Moderate evidence in the short and long term that MT for mixed acute and chronic LBP is similar for pain or disability to McKenzie therapy, general practice medical care, soft tissue therapy, PT, and education.

Study	Clients	Intervention and comparison (if any)	Outcome(s)
Utilization of thrust and nonthrust mobilization for low back pain: Grade B *(continued)*			
Slaven et al., 2013 (Level 1a)	8 studies of spine pain, including 2 studies of low back pain (260 participants)	Segment-specific level vs. nonspecific level spinal joint mobilization	Joint mobilization to the spine leads to an immediate effect on pain at rest and pain with the most painful movement. The direction of effect in the lumbar spine was toward nonspecific mobilization versus segment-specific mobilization.
Powers et al., 2008 (Level 2b)	30 adults (19 women), 18–45 years old	Posterior-anterior mobilization vs. a press-up exercise	There was a significant reduction in the average pain scores and increase in lumbar extension range of motion for both groups, supporting the use of posterior-anterior mobilization or a press-up exercise.
Utilization of thrust and nonthrust mobilization for sacroiliac joint syndrome: Grade D			
Kamali & Shokri, 2012 (Level 2b)	32 women	SIJ manipulation vs. SIJ manipulation + lumbar manipulation	Both groups showed significant improvements in pain and disability; however, SIJ + lumbar manipulation was more effective for improving disability than SIJ manipulation alone.

CLBP = chronic low back pain; LBP = low back pain; PT = physical therapy; MT = manual therapy; SIJ = sacroiliac joint; NSAIDs = nonsteroidal anti-inflammatory drugs

Mobilization and Manipulation of the Upper Extremity

Part III includes chapters on the shoulder, elbow, hand, and wrist. Chapter 7 covers various techniques for all joints of the shoulder, including sternoclavicular, acromioclavicular, glenohumeral, and scapulothoracic joints. In general, most pathology in the shoulder is at the glenohumeral joint, but the joints of the shoulder are so interconnected that knowing how to increase mobility in all of its joints is imperative for obtaining full function. Chapter 8 covers the 3 joints of the elbow—the humeroulnar, humeroradial, and proximal radioulnar joints. The joints of the elbow move primarily in flexion, extension, and forearm rotation. Chapter 9 covers the joints of the distal forearm, wrist, hand, and fingers.

Explicit instructions for all techniques are included with detailed overlaid photos to help the clinician with technique precision. The techniques described include multiple positions and potential modifications to accommodate clients who may have difficulty achieving a particular position. Current evidence for techniques is included in a table at the end of each chapter.

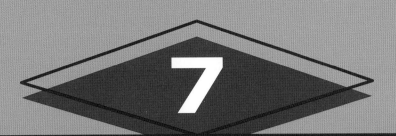

SHOULDER JOINT

LEARNING OBJECTIVES

After completing this chapter, you will be able to do the following:

- Describe the bony and soft tissue anatomy of the shoulder complex
- Identify the joint kinematics of the shoulder complex
- Describe positioning, movements, and reasoning behind shoulder mobilizations
- Identify evidence supportive of joint mobilization techniques for the shoulder

The shoulder joint is actually a complex arrangement of 4 different joints that work in unison to allow the largest range of motion of any joint in the body. Each joint in this complex is unique in its own right. Because of this complex interplay among joints, limitations of movement in one joint will create limitations in joints proximal or distal, resulting in shoulder dysfunction. It is therefore imperative to have a full understanding of the unique motions at each of these joints to provide optimal treatment to those with shoulder dysfunction.

Injuries that can cause a limitation of motion at the shoulder complex are many. Most injuries occur in or around the glenohumeral joint. Injuries at the glenohumeral joint can include labral tears, rotator cuff disease and tears, and capsular inflammation. Other injuries to the sternoclavicular joint or acromioclavicular joint can result from ligament sprains, whereas scapulothoracic joint injury is usually the result of overuse.

Anatomy

The shoulder is a complex articulation composed of multiple bones and synovial joints. It may be one of the most complex joints in the human body. Its 5 bones and 4 different articulations provide a substantial range of movement. The shoulder joint complex is comprised of the glenohumeral, acromioclavicular and sternoclavicular, and scapulothoracic joints. Each joint is unique, and a full understanding of the anatomy and kinematics of each joint is needed to properly treat the client with shoulder dysfunction.

Glenohumeral Joint

The glenohumeral joint (figure 7.1) is a multiaxial ball-and-socket synovial joint that allows a tremendous amount of movement through 3 degrees of freedom. The actual articulation occurs between a shallow concave glenoid fossa and a large convex humeral head. Static stabilization occurs through the glenohumeral ligaments, capsule, and the glenoid labrum, while dynamic stabilization occurs primarily through the rotator cuff muscles.

The glenohumeral joint has a large capsule and associated ligaments that cover approximately twice the surface area as that of the humeral head. This capsule is synovial lined and extends from the glenoid neck, or labrum, to the proximal shaft, or anatomical neck (figure 7.2) The ligaments that form the glenohumeral joint are the superior glenohumeral ligament (SGHL), the middle glenohumeral ligament (MGHL), and the inferior glenohumeral ligament complex (IGHLC). The SGHL runs from the superior portion of the labrum near the attachment of the long head of the biceps and from the base of the coracoid process and runs to the superior aspect of the humeral neck. The SGHL is taut when the arm is fully adducted near the side or when inferior translation occurs with the arm in a dependent position. The MGHL originates beneath the supraglenoid tubercle and the anterosuperior portion of the labrum and inserts just medial to the lessor tuberosity. The MGHL can resist an anteriorly directed force with the arm in an adducted position up to approximately 45° and limits extreme external rotations with the arm at the side. The IGHLC is a larger complex of ligament fibers that attach proximally along the anterior inferior rim of the glenoid fossa and to the glenoid labrum. Its distal attachment include the anterior and posterior inferior margins of the anatomical neck of the humerus. This complex has both anterior and posterior bands of ligaments that form a hammock of tissue between these bands. The IGHLC can resist several motions of the humerus. It becomes the primary resistance to inferior translation when the shoulder is abducted to 90°. Additionally, anterior and posterior translations can be resisted when the humerus is abducted to 90° and rotated either medially or laterally. When lateral rotation is added to the abducted position, the IGHLC resists anterior translation, while with internal rotation the IGHLC resists posterior translations.

Sternoclavicular Joint

The sternoclavicular joint (figure 7.3) is the only joint that actually links the upper extremity with the axial skeleton. This is a saddle-shaped diarthrodial synovial joint. Because of this saddle shape, the medial end of the clavicle and the sternum is inherently unstable. Between the 2 bony structures exists a cartilaginous articular disc that helps provide stability and cushions the joint. The sternoclavicular joint relies heavily on ligamentous support for stability. Ligaments include the anterior and posterior sternoclavicular ligaments, the costoclavicular ligaments, the interclavicular ligament, and the sternoclavicular joint capsule. Anterior and posterior clavicle restraint is provided by the anterior and posterior sternoclavicular ligament and the sternoclavicular joint capsule. Elevation of the clavicle is restricted by the costoclavicular ligament.

Acromioclavicular Joint

The acromioclavicular joint (figure 7.4) is a plane synovial joint located at the distal end of the clavicle and the acromion. The acromioclavicular joint is a plane diarthrodial synovial joint with 3 degrees of freedom. Between the 2 structures exists a fibrocartilaginous disc that varies in size. This joint has multiple ligaments to help provide static stability. The acromioclavicular joint has a capsule that surrounds the joint with additional ligamentous stabilization from the conoid and trapezoid ligaments that are medial to the joint proper. Anterior and posterior displacement is resisted by the acromioclavicular joint capsule. Depression of the acromion or elevation of the clavicle is resisted by the joint capsule and the conoid and trapezoid ligaments.

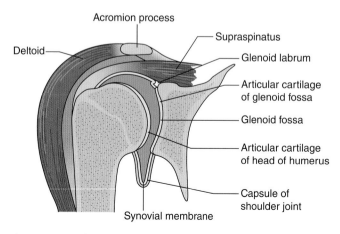

Figure 7.1 Glenohumeral joint.

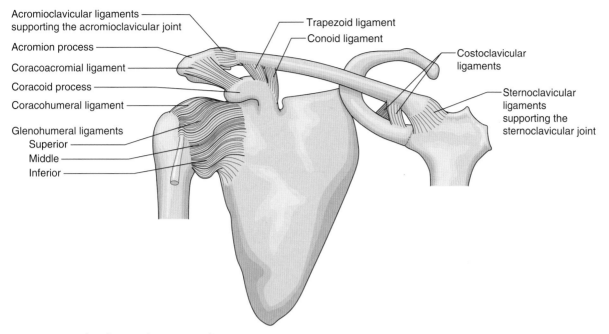

Figure 7.2 Glenohumeral joint capsule.

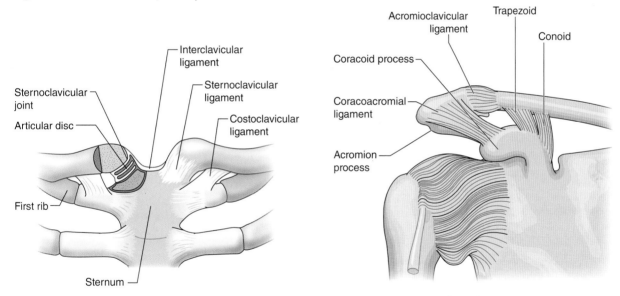

Figure 7.3 Sternoclavicular joint.

Figure 7.4 Acromioclavicular joint.

It is not uncommon following postsurgical procedures to the shoulder for the client to develop stiffness and associated pain. These injuries from rotator cuff repairs to labral repairs all require interruption of the joint capsule and associated structures. Due to injury, the joint is susceptible to irritation and inflammation. Restricted motion does not always resolve on its own as the repaired structures heal. It is important for the clinician to always assess joint passive mobility to ensure that the joint is allowing normal appropriate passive mobility.

Clinical Tips

Scapular dyskinesia is an abnormal movement of the scapular either at rest or during active movement of the shoulder. These abnormal movements can be caused by weakness of the scapular dynamic stabilizers. However, part of this altered pattern of movement can also include limited motion at the glenohumeral joint. Limited inferior and posterior capsular mobility may alter the normal scapulohumeral rhythm, resulting in early and faster scapular upward rotation during elevation. Inferior and posterior capsular mobility should always be assessed to ensure that normal mobility exists.

Scapulothoracic Joint

The scapulothoracic joint is considered a pseudojoint, as it does not have all the same characteristics of a normal synovial joint. This joint is a nonsynovial articulation between the broad, flat triangular scapula and the posterolateral aspect of the thorax and ribs.

Joint Kinematics

The shoulder joint has a complex array of movement patterns that require unique, yet characteristic joint kinematics. The joint kinematics described in the following sections are due to the joint bony surfaces, interposing cartilage structures, and surrounding soft tissues.

Glenohumeral

Movement of the glenohumeral joint occurs through 3 planes of motion. Shoulder flexion and extension occur around a mediolateral axis of rotation. Shoulder abduction and adduction occur around an anteroposterior axis. Internal and external rotations occur around a superoinferior axis.

Shoulder flexion occurs in the sagittal plane as a spinning of the joint along the glenoid face (figure 7.5). As long as the motion occurs in the sagittal plane, the glenohumeral joint does not require the rolling and gliding that occurs with other shoulder motions. Differing opinions report rotations during shoulder flexion. During elevation past 90°, there may be some slight internal rotation due to tightness of the coracohumeral ligament.

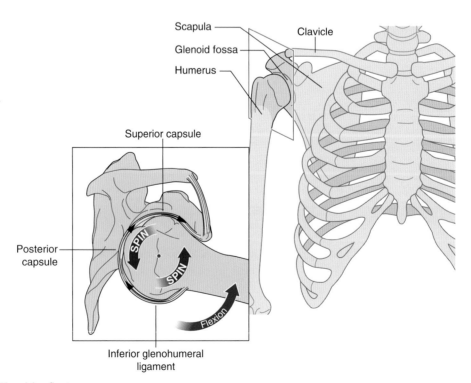

Figure 7.5 Shoulder flexion.

Shoulder extension would occur in the sagittal plane as a spinning of the joint on the glenoid face, opposite of that which occurs during shoulder flexion.

Shoulder external rotation occurs in the transverse plane through a superoinferior axis. As the humerus externally rotates, the convex humeral head rolls posteriorly (figure 7.6). Because the glenoid fossa is smaller than that of the humeral head, the humeral head will glide anteriorly while it rolls posteriorly so that it does not roll off the back of the glenoid fossa. Shoulder internal rotation occurs in the transverse plane through

a superoinferior axis. As the humerus moves into internal rotation, an anterior rolling of the convex humeral head occurs on the glenoid. During this anterior rolling, a posterior gliding occurs.

Shoulder abduction and adduction occur in the frontal plane around an anteroposterior axis. The center of rotation during abduction and adduction occurs through the center of the humeral head. As the convex humeral head rolls superior during abduction, there is a concomitant inferior glide motion (figure 7.7). During shoulder adduction, the humeral head rolls inferiorly as there is a superior gliding motion.

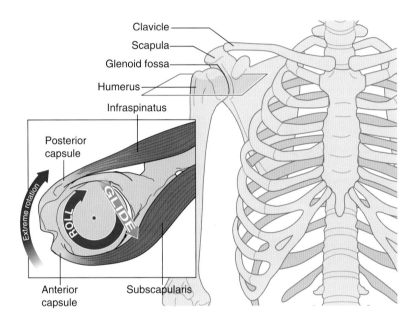

Figure 7.6   Shoulder external rotation.

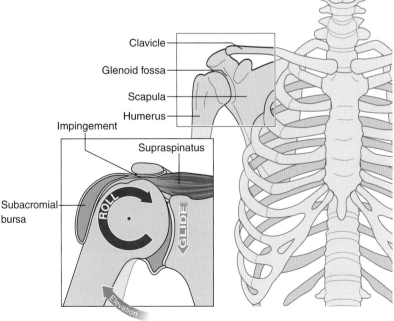

Figure 7.7   Shoulder abduction.

Sternoclavicular

The sternoclavicular joint is a saddle joint that allows 3 degrees of freedom. Typically, a saddle joint allows only 2 degrees of freedom, but there is a small amount of rotation that occurs at this joint also. Elevation and depression of the clavicle occur around an anteroposterior axis in the coronal plane. Protraction and retraction occur around a vertical axis in the transverse plane. Anterior and posterior rotations occur around a coronal axis in the sagittal plane.

Elevation of the sternoclavicular joint occurs between the convex medial clavicle and the con-

cave sternum. With elevation, the medial end of the clavicle rolls superiorly but depresses or glides inferiorly, as the lateral end of the clavicle elevates (figure 7.8). Depression occurs as the medial end of the clavicle rolls inferiorly and glides superiorly at the joint (figure 7.9).

Protraction occurs around a vertical axis along the transverse plane. The medial end of the clavicle is concave so that portion will roll and glide together anteriorly. During retraction, the concave medial end rolls and glides posteriorly (figure 7.10). The small amount of rotation that occurs at the sternoclavicular joint occurs around the

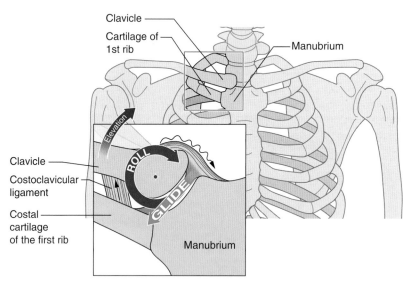

Figure 7.8 Clavicular elevation.

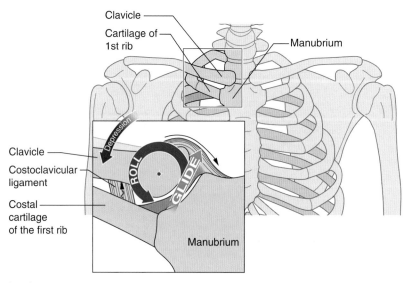

Figure 7.9 Clavicular depression.

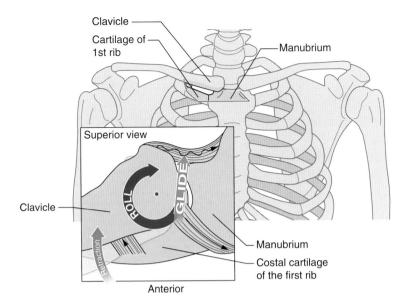

Figure 7.10 Shoulder retraction.

coronal axis in the sagittal plane. Rotations both anterior and posterior occur as a spinning of the medial clavicle along its long axis.

Acromioclavicular

The acromioclavicular joint is a plane synovial joint that allows upward and downward motions of the scapula and some anterior and posterior tipping. Motions of upward and downward rotation will occur in an oblique anteroposterior axis around the frontal plane, while the tipping motions will occur around an oblique coronal axis around the sagittal plane. Motions of internal and external rotation will occur at the acromioclavicular joint around a vertical axis in the transverse plane. The true arthrokinematics of the acromioclavicular joint are not widely discussed due to limited studies, all with inconsistent findings. We prefer to treat it as a plane joint with anterior and posterior gliding of one surface on the other.

Scapulothoracic

The scapulothoracic joint is not a true joint and therefore there is no arthrokinematic movement. However, we will describe mobilization procedures to help create more purposeful movement in those with stiffness and loss of scapular passive mobility. Passive motions at the scapular are as described within the primary motions (figure 7.11). The primary motions of the scapulothoracic joint movements are elevation and depression, upward and downward rotation, abduction and adduction, and internal and external rotation. Additional motions that are not typical in other joints but that occur at the scapulothoracic joint are tipping and winging.

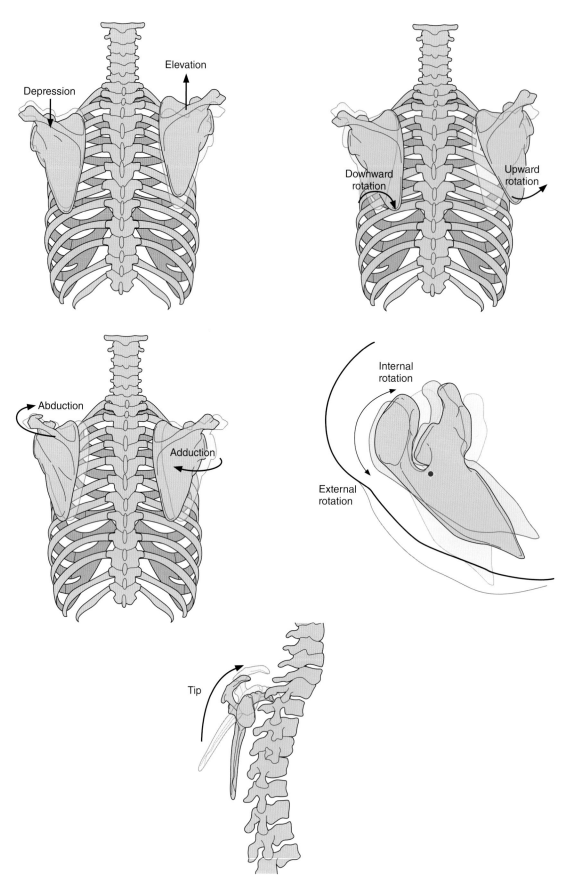

Figure 7.11 Scapulothoracic joint motions.

SHOULDER JOINT ARTHROLOGY

Articular surfaces	Closed packed position	Resting position	Capsular pattern	ROM norms	End-feel
Glenohumeral					
Glenoid: concave Humerus: convex	Full external rotation and full abduction	55°–70° abduction 30° horizontal adduction, neutral rotation	External rotation limited more than abduction limited more than internal rotation	Flexion = 180 Abduction = 180 Internal rotation = 70 External rotation = 90	Flexion = tissue stretch; abduction = bone-to-bone or tissue stretch; external rotation = tissue stretch; internal rotation = tissue stretch; extension = tissue stretch; adduction = tissue stretch; horizontal adduction = tissue stretch or soft tissue approximation; horizontal abduction = tissue stretch
Sternoclavicular					
Manubrium: concave proximal to distal (elevation/depression); convex ventral to dorsal (protraction/retraction) Clavicle: convex proximal to distal (elevation/depression); concave ventral to dorsal (protraction/retraction)	Maximal arm elevation	Clavicle horizontal, scapula 5 cm lateral to spinous process and superior angle of scapula at second rib while the inferior angle is at the seventh rib	Full elevation is limited	Elevation = 10–15 Protraction and retraction = 15–30 Posterior rotation = 15–31	Not described
Acromioclavicular					
Acromion: concave Clavicle: convex	Arm abducted to 90°	Clavicle horizontal, scapula 5 cm lateral to spinous process and superior angle of scapula at second rib while the inferior angle is at the seventh rib	Full elevation is limited	Upward rotation = 30 Downward rotation = 17	Not described
Scapulothoracic					
Thorax: convex Scapula: concave	None, not a true synovial joint	Clavicle horizontal, scapula 5 cm lateral to spinous process and superior angle of scapula at second rib while the inferior angle is at the seventh rib	None, not a true synovial joint	Not a true joint, so motion ranges not described	Not described

Distraction, Loose Packed Position

Client position: Supine with arm in 55° to 70° abduction in scapular plane and 30° flexion.

Clinician position: Standing, facing client's head.

Stabilization: Clinician grasps the proximal humerus from the medial and lateral sides. Client's hand is held between clinician's elbow and trunk.

Mobilization: Both hands will move the proximal humerus away from the glenoid joint surface at a 90° angle. The proximal humerus is moved in a lateral, ventral, and inferior direction.

Goal of technique: To increase general capsular mobility.

Note: This technique can be somewhat physically demanding.

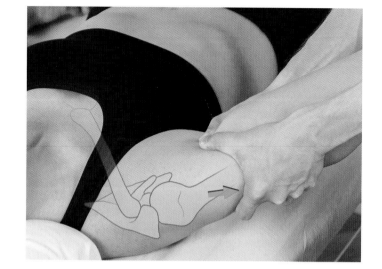

Lateral Distraction, in Flexion

Client position: Supine with humerus at 90° of shoulder flexion and slight horizontal adduction.

Clinician position: Standing alongside client's shoulder with proximal hand on the proximal humerus and distal hand stabilizing the humerus just proximal to elbow.

Stabilization: Client is stabilized by bodyweight on treatment table.

Mobilization: The humerus is laterally distracted away from the body in the frontal plane.

Goal of technique: To apply a very good stretch to the superior and posterior capsule.

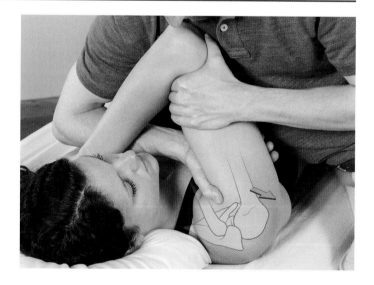

Notes: The clinician can apply an internal or external rotation to selectively tighten or loosen the posterior capsule to desired level. The clinician can also mobilize in a caudal direction to stretch the inferior capsule.

Inferior Glide, Loose Packed, Supine

VIDEO 7.1 **in the web study guide shows this technique.**

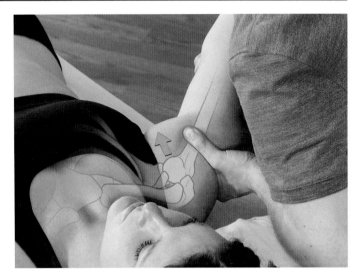

Client position: Supine with the humerus in 55° to 70° abduction and 30° of flexion.

Clinician position: Standing alongside client shoulder toward head, turned to face feet.

Stabilization: Clinician's proximal hand contacts the proximal portion of client's superior humerus, while distal hand stabilizes humerus directly above elbow.

Mobilization: The humeral head is glided inferior, anterior, and slightly laterally.

Goal of technique: To treat accessory motion restriction for glenohumeral elevation.

Note: Some slight lateral distraction might be needed because of the inclination of the glenoid fossa.

Inferior Glide, Loose Packed, Sitting

Client position: Seated upright with support as needed for distal extremity on treatment table. The glenohumeral joint should be near 55° of abduction and 30° of flexion.

Clinician position: Alongside and behind client's shoulder to be mobilized.

Stabilization: Proximal hand contacts over the superior proximal humeral head with one (pictured) or both hands. The distal humerus will be controlled with use of leg or table for stabilization.

Mobilization: With arm in slight abduction, pressure is applied to the humerus inferiorly and slightly anteriorly to elicit a gliding motion.

Goal of technique: To treat accessory motion restriction for glenohumeral elevation.

Note: This is a great mobilization because of the excellent mechanical advantage for the clinician and ability for good relaxation from the client.

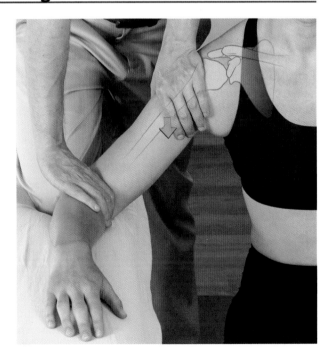

Inferior Glide, End ROM, Sitting

Client position: Sitting, with glenohumeral joint in scaption or abduction to the first noticed motion barrier.

Clinician position: Standing behind client, facing the glenohumeral joint to be treated, one hand wrapped over the proximal humerus.

Stabilization: Distal humerus rests with elbow on treatment table for stabilization (as shown).

Mobilization: A downward pressure is applied to the humeral head to elicit an inferiorly, anteriorly, and slightly lateral gliding motion.

Goal of technique: To treat accessory motion restriction for glenohumeral elevation.

Note: This technique affords good mechanical advantage for the clinician.

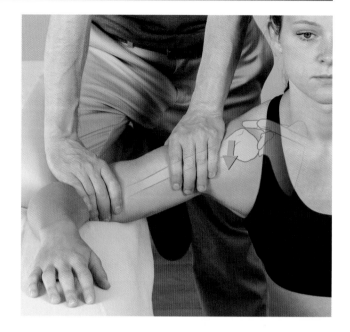

Anterior Glide, Loose Packed Position, Supine

Client position: Supine, with the arm in 55° to 70° of abduction in scapular plane and 30° of flexion.

Clinician position: Facing client's head from a caudal direction.

Stabilization: Grasping the posterior aspect of proximal humerus, with thumbs located on the anterior surface of proximal humerus. Client's distal arm is stabilized with clinician's arm closest to client's body.

Mobilization: Pressure is placed on the humeral head to glide it in the anterior and medial direction parallel to the surface of the glenoid fossa or perpendicular to the plane of the scapula.

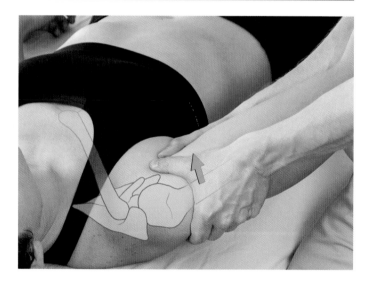

Goal of technique: To treat accessory motion of anterior glide for restrictions in glenohumeral external rotation.

Notes: Scapular stabilization is greatly compromised when mobilizing in this position when using higher grade III or grade IV mobilizations. The use of a belt or assistant to stabilize client may be helpful. This mobilization can be performed in various degrees of glenohumeral abduction.

Anterior Glide, Loose Packed Position, Prone

Client position: Prone, arm in loose packed position. May need towel roll under coracoid process for comfort.

Clinician position: Standing facing client's head from a caudal direction.

Stabilization: Distal hand holds humerus slightly above client's elbow joint.

Mobilization: The proximal hand contacts client's shoulder along the proximal humerus as close to the joint line as possible. Pressure is applied to the posterior humeral head to glide it in an anterior and medial direction, parallel to the surface of the glenoid fossa.

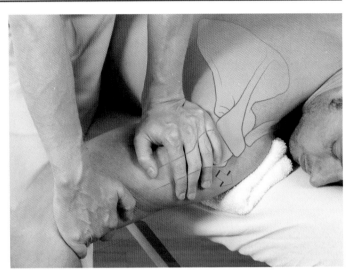

Goal of technique: To treat accessory motion of anterior glide for restrictions in glenohumeral external rotation.

Notes: The prone position allows for greater scapular stabilization, since the scapular is blocked in this position by the treatment table. The clinician may also apply a slight distraction force to the humerus prior to mobilizing to take up capsular slack. This technique can be performed in various degrees of shoulder abduction.

Anterior Capsule/Soft Tissue Physiological Mobilization

Client position: Supine, with the affected arm in loose packed position or higher degrees of elevation if possible. Only the distal humerus and elbow are off the edge of the mobilization table.

Clinician position: Standing facing client's head from a caudal direction.

Stabilization: Stabilization of client is through bodyweight imparted to the treatment table.

Mobilization: Arm is taken through full available range of motion of shoulder external rotation with oscillations performed at the available end range of motion.

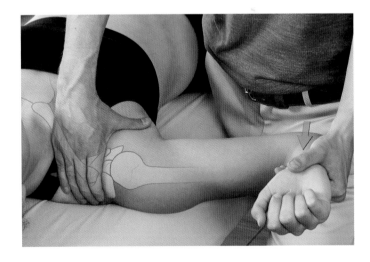

Goal of technique: To increase overall physiological range of motion of glenohumeral external rotation.

Anterior Glide With Combination of External Shoulder Rotation and Shoulder Abduction

Client position: Prone with shoulder abducted in frontal plane to end point and external rotation at end point.

Clinician position: Standing facing client's head with leg elevated enough to stabilize client's distal humerus on knee. Client's forearm will rest on clinician's knee.

Stabilization: The manipulating hand contacts posterior proximal humerus while stabilizing hand helps hold client's distal humerus in place. The stabilizing hand can also assist in fine-tuning position of humerus.

Mobilization: Pressure is applied to the posterior humerus to glide in an anterior and medial direction parallel to surface of the glenoid fossa.

Goal of technique: To treat accessory motion of anterior glide for restrictions in glenohumeral external rotation.

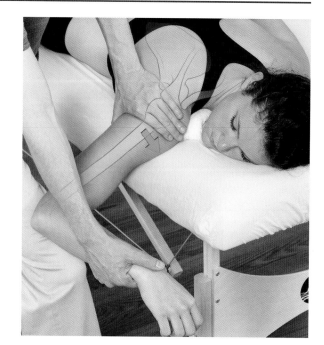

Notes: This is an advanced position and should be used cautiously. This is best used with higher grades of mobilizations, such as III and IV.

Posterior (Dorsal) Glide, in Adduction

Client position: Supine, with arm near side between clinician's arm and trunk with the glenohumeral joint in a neutral rotation.

Clinician position: Standing facing client from a caudal position.

Stabilization: Proximal hand contacts the anterior humerus, while other hand stabilizes the distal humerus and the treatment table stabilizes the scapula. Client's hand should be held between clinician's arm and trunk.

Mobilization: Pressure is applied to the anterior humeral head, imparting a laterally and posteriorly directed gliding motion parallel to the glenoid fossa.

Goal of technique: To treat accessory motion of posterior glide for restrictions in glenohumeral internal rotation and forward flexion.

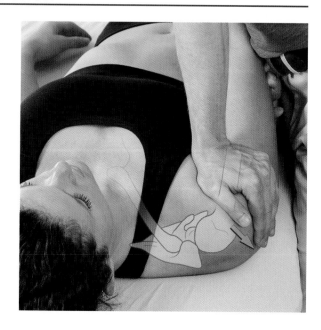

Notes: This is a very comfortable technique. Clinician can add glenohumeral internal rotation to impart more of a stretch on the posterior capsule.

Posterior Glide, in Loose Packed Position

Client position: Supine, glenohumeral joint in 55° to 70° of abduction and 30° of flexion.

Clinician position: Standing facing client's head from a caudal position.

Stabilization: Distal hand controls the distal humerus above the elbow. Client's hand held between clinician's elbow and trunk.

Mobilization: Proximal hand contacts the anterior proximal humerus as pressure is applied to create a lateral and posterior glide to the humeral head.

Goal of technique: To treat accessory motion of posterior glide for restrictions in glenohumeral internal rotation and forward flexion.

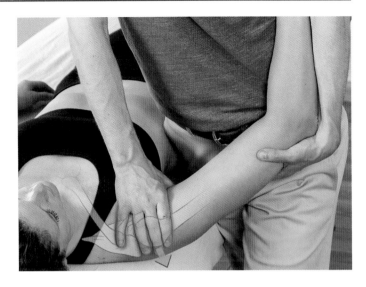

Note: The supine position affords good scapular stability.

Posterior Glide, in Flexion

> *VIDEO 7.2* **in the web study guide shows this technique.**

Client position: Supine, humerus in 90° of flexion, slight horizontal adduction medial to the sagittal plane, elbow flexed 90°.

Clinician position: Standing facing client's head from a caudal position.

Stabilization: Distal hand is placed over client's elbow, while proximal hand stabilizes the posterior portion of the scapula.

Mobilization: Clinician's body provides a posterior-lateral directed pressure through the long axis of the humerus, imparting a posterior and lateral gliding movement of the humeral head.

Goal of technique: To treat accessory motion of posterior glide for restrictions in internal rotation and forward flexion.

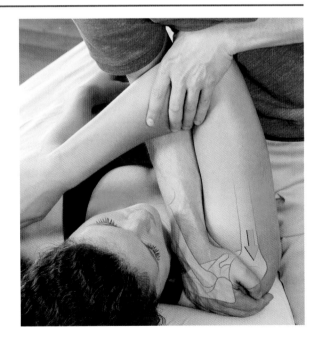

Note: The clinician can add humeral internal rotation to increase the effect of the mobilization.

Posterior Capsule/Soft Tissue Physiological Mobilization

Client position: Supine, with arm in 90°abduction and 90° elbow flexion. Only the distal humerus and elbow are off the edge of the mobilization table.

Clinician position: Standing superior or cephalad to the client, facing client's head.

Stabilization: Proximal arm stabilizes the scapula by applying force across the deltopectoral groove from clinician's forearm.

Mobilization: Glenohumeral joint is taken through full available range of motion of glenohumeral internal rotation, with oscillations performed at the end of the available range of motion.

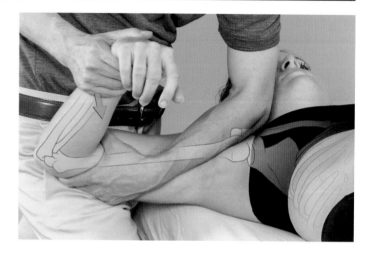

Goal of technique: To increase overall physiological range of motion of internal rotation and help with forward flexion.

Note: This is an excellent mobilization to gain purely glenohumeral internal rotation.

Dorsal Glide

VIDEO 7.3 **in the web study guide shows this technique.**

Client position: Supine, with arm neutral in comfortable position.

Clinician position: Standing slightly caudal, facing client's head, on the affected side on which the mobilization is to be performed.

Stabilization: No stabilization required. Bodyweight will keep client in correct position.

Mobilization: The thumb pad is used over the anterior sternal end of the clavicle approximately 3 cm from most medial portion. A second thumb is used to gently oscillate the clavicle in the posterior direction.

Goal of technique: To treat accessory motion of posterior glide for restrictions in clavicle retraction.

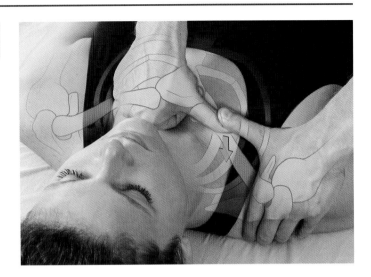

Ventral Glide

Client position: Supine, with arm neutral in comfortable position.

Clinician position: Standing, slightly caudal, facing client's head, on the side on which the mobilization is to be performed.

Stabilization: Over client's sternum.

Mobilization: The manipulating hand grasps around the clavicle to the ventral surface with the fingers. While stabilizing hand holds the sternum, manipulating hand glides the clavicle in a ventral direction.

Goal of technique: To treat accessory motion of anterior glide for restrictions in clavicle protraction.

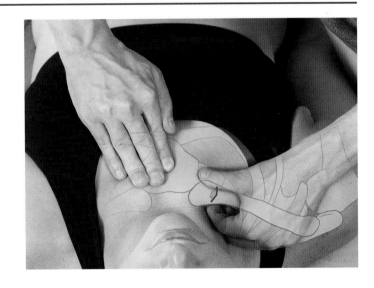

Note: It might be difficult with this technique to get a good grasp of the clavicle due to muscle spasm, mass, or tightness.

Cranial Glide

Client position: Supine, arm supported in relaxed position.

Clinician position: Standing, slightly caudal, facing client's head, on the side on which the mobilization is to be performed.

Stabilization: No stabilization required.

Mobilization: Thumb is placed over the inferior portion of the proximal clavicle about 3 cm lateral to the most medial aspect. The clavicle is mobilized superiorly and medially, parallel to the sternal articular surface.

Goal of technique: To treat accessory motion of superior glide for restrictions in clavicle depression.

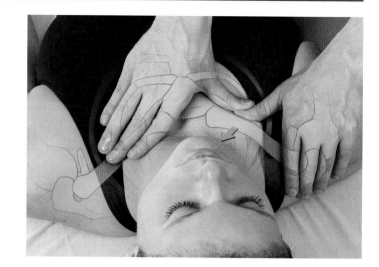

Note: This technique can also be used to assist shoulder girdle depression.

Caudal Glide

 VIDEO 7.4 in the web study guide shows this technique.

Client position: Supine, in a relaxed position.

Clinician position: Standing from a cephalad position, facing client's head.

Stabilization: No stabilization required.

Mobilization: Either thumb is placed over the superior portion of the proximal clavicle about 3 cm lateral to the most medial aspect. Pressure is applied through the thumb to the clavicle to mobilize in an inferior and lateral direction.

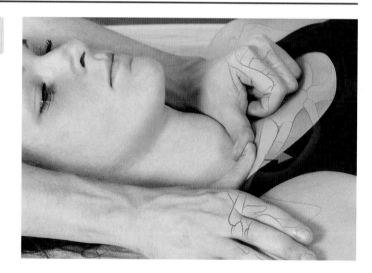

Goal of technique: To treat accessory motion of inferior glide for restrictions in clavicle elevation.

Dorsal Glide

VIDEO 7.5 **in the web study guide shows this technique.**

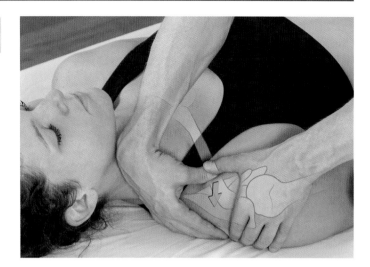

Client position: Sitting or supine, arm in relaxed position.

Clinician position: Standing beside client on side to be mobilized.

Stabilization: Proximal hand contacts distal clavicle with thumb placed anterior while index finger pad is placed on the posterior surface. Distal hand stabilizes the scapula with the index finger on the posterior acromion of the scapula.

Mobilization: May use thumb-over-thumb technique if more comfortable. A posterior glide is imparted to the distal clavicle to create a dorsal gliding motion.

Goal of technique: To increase joint play and mobility in acromioclavicular joint.

Note: Performance of this mobilization in seated position does not allow for very good scapular stabilization.

Dorsal Glide—Method 2

Client position: Best performed with client sitting.

Clinician position: Standing alongside client on the side of affected shoulder.

Stabilization: Hand is placed over the dorsolateral surface of the scapular along the posterior acromion and the distal scapular spine.

Mobilization: The manipulating hand contacts the clavicle via the thenar or hypothenar eminence to glide the clavicle in a dorsal direction.

Goal of technique: To increase joint play and mobility in acromioclavicular joint.

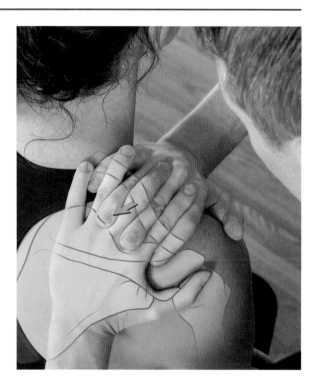

Ventral Glide

 VIDEO 7.6 **in the web study guide shows this technique.**

Client position: Best performed with client sitting.

Clinician position: Standing behind the client.

Stabilization: Fingers are placed along the anterior acromion and over the ventral surface of the proximal humerus.

Mobilization: The thumb-over-thumb technique is used by the manipulating hand to impart pressure to glide the clavicle in a ventral direction.

Goal of technique: To increase joint play and mobility in acromioclavicular joint.

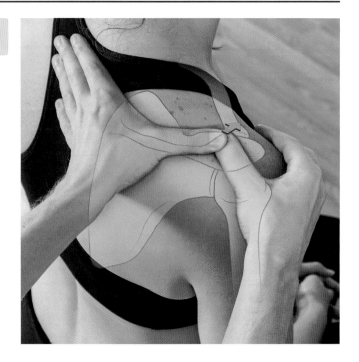

Distraction

VIDEO 7.7 in the web study guide shows this technique.

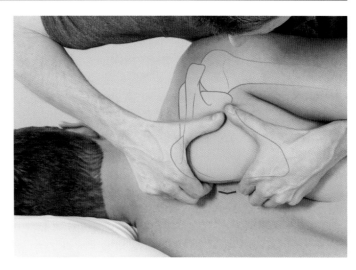

Client position: Side-lying at edge of treatment table, ventral side of body facing clinician, glenohumeral joint in adduction.

Clinician position: At front of treatment table facing client.

Stabilization: Anterior portion of the shoulder is held against clinician's delto-pectoral groove for added leverage.

Mobilization: Both hands grasp the medial border of the posterior scapula. The medial border of the scapula is gently separated from the posterior thorax. A sustained hold or intermittent stretch can be used to decrease muscular resistance. An alternate method is to slide mobilizing hand under inferior medial angle of scapula and distract from this position, while superior hand stabilizes scapula over the acromioclavicular joint.

Goal of technique: To treat overall restrictions of scapular mobility.

Note: Once the client is relaxed, you might add other components, such as medial or lateral rotation, protraction/retraction, and so on.

Cranial Glide

Client position: Side-lying at edge of treatment table, ventral side of body facing clinician, glenohumeral joint in adduction.

Clinician position: At front of treatment table facing client.

Stabilization: Bodyweight of client will stabilize.

Mobilization: The manipulating hand is placed over the inferior angle of the posterior scapula. The guiding hand is positioned over the acromion. Manipulating hand glides the scapula superiorly in a cranial direction, while guiding hand controls and stabilizes the scapula.

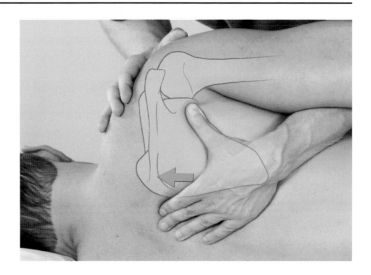

Goal of technique: To treat restrictions of scapular elevation.

Caudal Glide

Client position: Side-lying at edge of treatment table, ventral side of body facing clinician, glenohumeral joint in adduction.

Clinician position: At front of treatment table facing client.

Stabilization: Bodyweight of client will stabilize.

Mobilization: The manipulating hand is over the acromioclavicular joint, while the guiding hand is positioned over the posterior inferior angle of the scapula. Manipulating hand will glide the acromion in a caudal direction, while guiding hand controls and stabilizes the scapula.

Goal of technique: To treat restrictions of scapular depression.

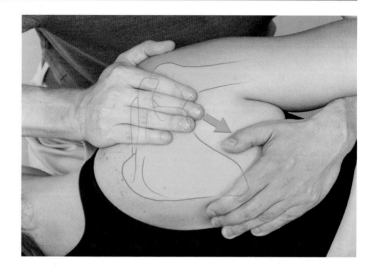

Lateral Glide

Client position: Side-lying at edge of treatment table, ventral side of body facing clinician, glenohumeral joint in adduction.

Clinician position: At front of treatment table facing client.

Stabilization: Bodyweight of client will stabilize.

Mobilization: Both clinician's hands are positioned with fingertips over the posterior vertebral border of the scapula. Both hands gently glide the scapula in a lateral direction.

Goal of technique: To treat restrictions of scapular lateral glide.

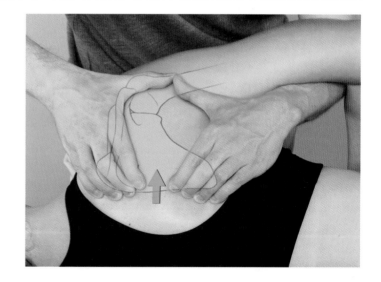

Medial Glide

Client position: Side-lying at edge of treatment table, ventral side of body facing clinician, the glenohumeral joint in adduction.

Clinician position: At front of treatment table facing client.

Stabilization: Bodyweight of client will stabilize.

Mobilization: Both hands will be positioned over the posterior-lateral border of the scapula—one over the acromion, and the other over the lower axillary border. Both hands gently glide the scapula in a medial direction.

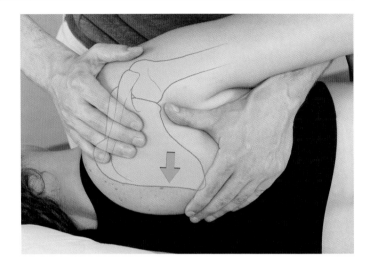

Goal of technique: To treat restrictions of scapular medial glide.

Lateral Rotation

Client position: Side-lying at edge of treatment table, ventral side of body facing clinician, glenohumeral joint in adduction.

Clinician position: At front of treatment table facing client.

Stabilization: None required. Bodyweight of client will stabilize.

Mobilization: Both clinician's hands are positioned with fingertips over the posterior vertebral border of the scapula. Both hands gently glide the scapula in the direction of lateral rotation.

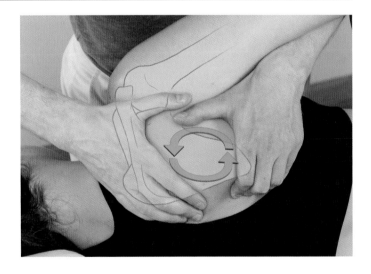

Goal of technique: To treat restrictions of scapular lateral rotation glide.

Medial Rotation

Client position: Side-lying at the edge of treatment table, ventral side of body facing clinician, glenohumeral joint in adduction.

Clinician position: At front of treatment table facing client.

Stabilization: Bodyweight of client will stabilize.

Mobilization: Both clinician's hands are positioned with fingertips over the posterior vertebral border of the scapula. Both hands gently glide the scapula in the direction of medial rotation.

Goal of technique: To treat restrictions of scapular medial rotation glide.

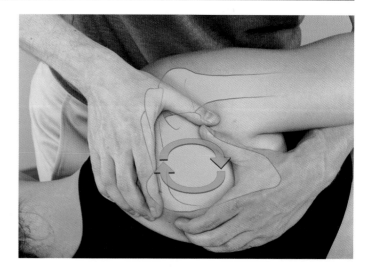

Go to the web study guide and complete the case study for this chapter. The case study discusses an 18-year-old competitive high school swimmer with shoulder pain and limited motion following capsular plication.

EVIDENCE FOR MANUAL THERAPY OF VARIOUS SHOULDER JOINT PATHOLOGIES

Study	Clients	Intervention and comparison (if any)	Outcome(s)
Utilization of mobilization for general shoulder conditions: Grade A			
Camarinos and Marinko, 2010 Systematic review (Level 1a)	7 studies	MT or reduction of pain, improving function, and increasing range of motion Comparing effects of different types of manual therapy on pain and quality of life	MT has a positive impact on functional movement in clients with shoulder pain. MT found a trend toward decreasing some measures of pain, and found significant within-group differences in improving quality of life. Overall recommendation from study: Studies demonstrate the benefit of MT for improvements in mobility and a trend in improving pain measures, while increasing in function and quality of life need further study.
Utilization of mobilization or manipulation for rotator cuff tendinopathy: Grade B			
Desjardins-Charbonneau et al., 2015 Systematic review and meta-analysis (Level 2b)	21 studies	MT alone vs control MT + exercise vs multimodal rehabilitation MT + other interventions vs multimodal rehabilitation	Significant effect in favor of MT. Magnitude of treatment effect is small but could be considered clinically important. Significant difference was observed for the addition of MT to exercise for overall pain reduction at 4 weeks. Magnitude of treatment effect is small but could be considered clinically important. High heterogeneity between trials prevented pooling of data. Overall recommendation from study: For clients with rotator cuff tendinopathy, based on low- to moderate-quality evidence, MT may decrease pain; however, it is unclear whether it can improve function.
Gebremariam et al., 2014 Literature review (Level 5)	10 studies; 2 reviews	Data extraction to summarize best evidence Effectiveness of joint mobilization Effectiveness of MT	Conflicting evidence for effectiveness of mobilization as an add-on therapy to exercise versus exercise alone. Limited evidence for the effectiveness of MT plus self-training alone in the short term.

(continued)

Study	Clients	Intervention and comparison (if any)	Outcome(s)
Utilization of mobilization and manipulation for adhesive capsulitis: Grade C			
Noten et al., 2016 (Level 5)	12 trials	Evaluated efficacy of mobilization technique on range of motion and pain in adults with adhesive capsulitis	Seven types of mobilization evaluated. Angular mobilization (2), Cyriax approach (1), and Maitland technique (6) showed improvement in pain and ROM. Posterior translational mobilization is preferred to increase external rotation. Spine mobilizations combined with glenohumeral stretching and both angular and translational mobilizations had superior effect on active ROM compared with sham ultrasound. High intensity mobilization showed less improvement than neglect. Positive long-term effects of Mulligan technique were found on both pain and ROM.
Page et al., 2014 (Level 5)	32 trials	Compared MT + exercise vs other interventions	Best available evidence show that combination of MT + exercise may not be as effective as glucocorticoid injection in short term. Unclear whether MT + exercise + electrotherapy is an effective adjunct to glucocorticoid injection or oral NSAID. MT + exercise following joint distention may confer similar to those of sham ultrasound but provide greater client-reported treatment success and active range of motion.

MT = manual therapy; ROM = range of motion; NSAID = nonsteroidal anti-inflammatory drug

ELBOW JOINT

LEARNING OBJECTIVES

After completing this chapter, you will be able to do the following:

- Describe the bony and soft tissue anatomy of the elbow complex
- Describe the joint kinematics of the elbow joint
- Describe positioning, movements, and reasoning behind elbow mobilization
- Identify evidence supporting joint mobilization techniques for the elbow

The elbow joint allows flexion and extension and supination and pronation of the forearm. These motions are very important for activities of daily living, including eating, grooming, and personal hygiene. These functions are performed via 3 different joints that make up the elbow complex. Limitations of motion in 1 joint can significantly affect the overall function of the entire joint. It is important therefore to fully understand the structure of each joint.

Anatomy

The elbow complex is composed of 3 joints: humeroradial, humeroulnar, and proximal radioulnar (figure 8.1). Multiple muscles provide dynamic movement of these joints. Each joint is unique in and of itself and will be described in more detail in the following sections.

Humeroulnar Joint

The joint that allows the greatest range of motion at the elbow is the humeroulnar joint. This joint is comprised of the distal portion of the humerus and the proximal ulna. Because this joint has a large amount of surface area of contact, a significant amount of motion occurs here. The primary motion that occurs at the humeroulnar joint is elbow flexion and extension. This motion occurs as the trochlea of the proximal ulna glides along the trochlear notch of the distal humerus.

Humeroradial Joint

The humeroradial joint is the articulation between the capitulum of the distal humerus and the proximal radius. This is a diarthrodial sellar joint that has very little contact between surfaces when the forearm is fully extended. During dynamic elbow flex-

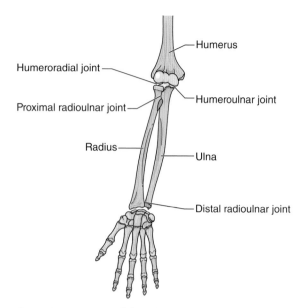

Figure 8.1 Joints of the elbow complex.

ion motion, the forearm muscles create a dynamic compressive effect approximating the joint surfaces. This joint participates in flexion and extension as well as rotation via supination and pronation.

Radioulnar Joint

There are 2 radioulnar joints, 1 proximal and 1 distal. The proximal joint is formed by the proxi-

mal end of the radius and the proximal ulna. This joint is formed where the radial notch of the ulna meets with the head of the radius. The head of the radius is held in place by the annular ligament that surrounds it via attachments both anterior and posterior on the ulna. The distal radioulnar joint is formed by the head of the ulna and the ulnar notch of the radius and will be discussed in the wrist and hand chapter.

Muscles

Muscles supply the elbow with flexion and extension and supination and pronation. These active motions are necessary to perform activities of daily living and play a critical role in sport and occupational movement.

Elbow and Forearm Flexors

The elbow flexors include biceps brachii, brachialis, and brachioradialis, while the forearm flexors include flexor carpi radialis and ulnaris, palmaris longus, and flexor digitorum superficialis (figure 8.2). The biceps is a large muscle that crosses both the glenohumeral and elbow joints and runs along the anterior elbow. The biceps has a large cross-sectional area and has a good mechanical advantage because it passes close to the axis of

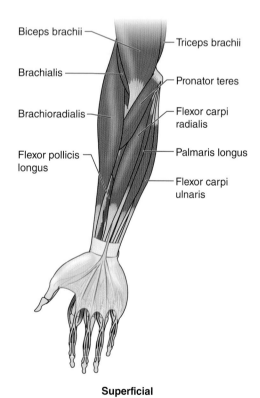

Superficial

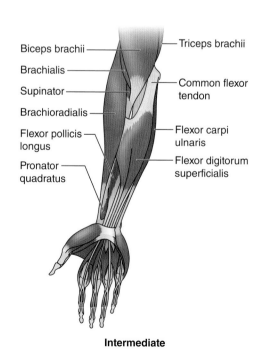

Intermediate

Figure 8.2 Elbow flexor and forearm flexor muscles.

rotation. The biceps brachii has 2 origins, including the supraglenoid tubercle of the scapula and the coracoid process. The biceps inserts onto the radial tuberosity. Because of its attachment on the radius, the biceps works best in conjunction with forearm supination.

The brachialis is a single-joint muscle that originates on the distal aspect of the anterior humerus and inserts onto the coronoid process and tuberosity of the proximal ulna. The brachialis is known to contract in all positions of forearm placement. The brachioradialis is a long narrow muscle that runs from the distal humerus to the radial styloid of the distal forearm.

The flexor carpi radialis originates from the common flexor tendon at the medial epicondyle and inserts distally near the radial side of the distal forearm at the base of the second and sometimes third metacarpal. It functions as a wrist flexor and does not act on the elbow. The flexor carpi ulnaris originates from the common flexor tendon at the medial epicondyle and inserts distally on the ulnar side of the forearm at the pisiform. The palmaris longus, if present, arises from the medial epicondyle and runs distally and inserts into the palmar aponeurosis. The flexor digitorum superficialis, similar to the other flexors, originates on the common flexor tendon and runs distally to attach to the base of the proximal interphalangeal joints.

Elbow and Forearm Extensors

The elbow and forearm extensors include the triceps brachii and the anconeus, while the forearm extensors include extensor carpi radialis longus, brevis, extensor digitorum communis, and extensor carpi ulnaris (figure 8.3). The triceps brachii fills the entire posterior surface of the humerus. The triceps brachii has 3 heads. The long head has its origin from the infraglenoid tubercle of the scapula. The lateral head originates from the proximal lateral intramuscular septum of the humerus. The medial head originates from the entire distal half of the posteromedial surface of the humerus. All of the heads converge as a common tendon that attaches to the tip of the olecranon process. The anconeus is a small muscle that originates on the lateral epicondyle and lateral triceps fascia and inserts into the dorsal proximal ulna.

The extensor carpi radialis longus originates from the supracondylar bony column below the origin of the brachioradialis and inserts into the base of the second metacarpal. The extensor carpi radialis brevis originates from the lateral epicondyle and inserts into the dorsal base of the third

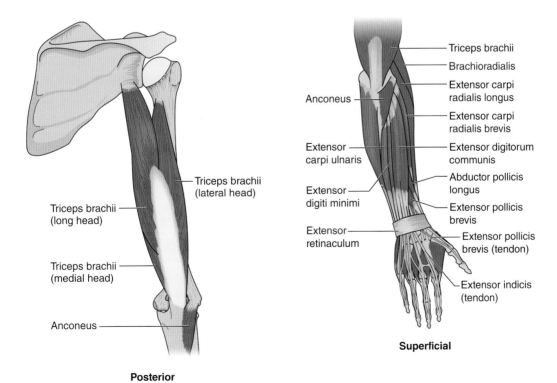

Posterior

Superficial

Figure 8.3 Elbow extensor and forearm extensor muscles.

Clinical Tip

Cadaveric studies (Lin et al., 2017; Park and Ahmad, 2004) have demonstrated that within the flexor-pronator mass, the flexor carpi ulnaris provides the most significant contribution to resisting valgus stress at the elbow.

---

metacarpal. The extensor digitorum communis arises from the anterior distal aspect of the lateral epicondyle and runs distally to insert into all fingers. Last, the extensor carpi ulnaris originates from 2 heads at the lateral epicondyle and inserts distally into the base of the fifth metacarpal.

Supinators and Pronators

The forearm supinator and pronator teres muscles rotate the forearm in the transverse plane. The supinator muscle originates from 3 sites: the lateral anterior aspect of the lateral epicondyle, the lateral collateral ligament, and the proximal anterior crest of the ulna. It runs distally, obliquely, and radially to attach at the proximal radius. The supinator is a weaker supinator than the biceps brachii, but because it does not cross the elbow joint, its strength is not altered by elbow flexion. The pronator teres has 2 heads, 1 of which originates from the anterosuperior aspect of the medial epicondyle and the second from the coronoid process of the ulna. The muscles run distally and insert at the proximal and middle portions of the radius into the tuberosity on its lateral aspect. Because it crosses the elbow joint it is a strong pronator and also a weak elbow flexor. See figure 8.2 for the pronator teres and supinator muscles.

Joint Capsule

The elbow joint capsule is large and extensive, covering all 3 elbow joints. It needs to be fairly large to allow such a great extent of movement—up to 150° of elbow flexion range of motion. The anterior portion of the capsule inserts proximally above the radial fossa and the coronoid, and attaches to the anterior margin of the coronoid medially and to the annular ligament laterally. The capsule attaches posteriorly just above the olecranon fossa and distally along the supracondylar columns. The capsule is relatively thin, but has thickenings both anteriorly and medially and laterally provided by attachments of the oblique and collateral ligaments along their respective locations. The anterior portion of the capsule is taut in extension, while the posterior portion is taut in flexion. As it is a synovial capsule, it is lined with a synovial membrane, which helps secrete synovial fluid to lubricate the joint for efficient movement.

Ligaments

Ligaments are designed to connect one bone to another and are important for structure support and stabilization. The elbow joint has several ligaments (figure 8.4) and membranes that help with maintenance of joint stability. These ligaments are specially formed as thickenings of the joint capsule.

◆ *Medial collateral ligament.* The medial collateral ligament is also called the ulnar collateral ligament (UCL) because of its attachment to the proximal ulna on the medial portion of the coronoid process. The UCL is composed of 3 bands. The anterior band provides most restraint to valgus forces at the elbow and is therefore the strongest. Most of the anterior bands' fibers become taut with elbow extension. The posterior band runs from the medial epicondyle to the medial side of the olecranon process. Its fibers become tight with increased elbow flexion. The oblique band attaches to both the anterior and posterior bands, just described, and therefore provides little stability.

◆ *Lateral collateral ligament.* Because of its location on the lateral side of the elbow the lateral collateral ligament is also called the radial collateral ligament (RCL). This ligament runs from the lateral epicondyle to the annular ligament and to the crest of the ulna. The RCL has several bundles, including the RCL proper, the annular ligament, and an oblique cord. This ligament restrains elbow varus and is taut throughout motion from flexion to extension indicating that its origin is very near the axis of rotation.

◆ *Annular ligament.* The annular ligament encircles the radial head and attaches to the anterior

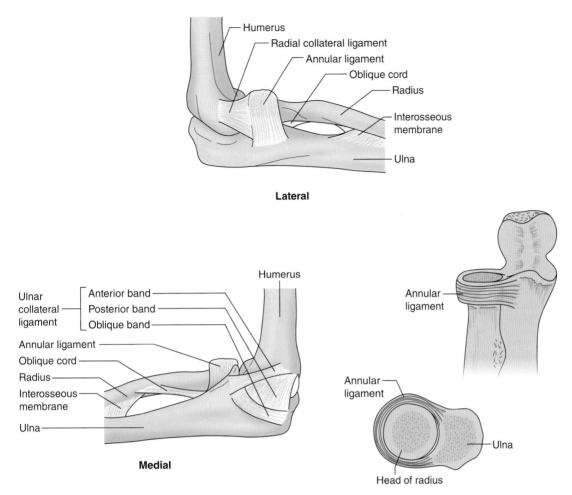

Figure 8.4 Major ligaments of the elbow.

and posterior portion of the lessor sigmoid notch. This ligament blends into the RCL. That anterior portion of the ligament becomes tight with supination while the posterior aspect becomes taut during pronation.

◆ *Quadrate ligament.* The quadrate ligament is a thin fibrous layer that covers the capsule and attaches along the inferior aspect of the radial notch to the neck of the radius. The anterior portion of the ligament stabilizes the joint during full supination. The posterior portion stabilizes the joint in full pronation.

◆ *Oblique cord.* The oblique cord runs from the inferior radial notch to the inferior aspect of the bicipital tuberosity. This ligament resists distal migration of the radius. It also becomes taut in full supination. This is a small ligament that may not be of great value.

Bursae

Several bursae exist in the elbow joint. The bursae are synovial-filled sacs that provide cushion and allow for reduced friction during joint movement. One of the biggest of the bursae is the subcutaneous (olecranon) bursa. This bursa, located between the olecranon process and the soft tissues that overlie it, is commonly injured. Other bursae include the intra-tendinous bursa, the subtendinous bursa, and the bicipitoradial bursae.

Joint Kinematics

This section will describe joint kinematics related to axes of motion, as well as arthrokinematics of the elbow joint. Each of the joints of the elbow will be individually discussed, but it must be remembered that all 3 of these joints work in unison with one another for full unrestricted elbow motion. The elbow joint kinematics described here are due to the joint bony surfaces, interposing articular cartilage, and surrounding soft tissues.

Humeroulnar

The humeroulnar joint moves the elbow into flexion and extension. The arthrokinematics of the humeroulnar joint occur as a sliding or gliding of the concave trochlear notch of the ulna along the convex articular surface of the trochlea of the distal humerus (figure 8.5). These motions almost always occur as an open kinetic chain movement. However, there are some instances such as during a pull-up or pushup exercise in which the arthrokinematic motions are reversed and the convex surface of the humerus may roll and glide in opposite directions as they move along a fixed concave surface of the proximal ulna.

Humeroradial

The humeroradial joint moves in flexion and extension. The arthrokinematics of this joint are a sliding and gliding of the concave fovea of the radial head against the convex capitulum of the distal humerus.

As the elbow is moved into flexion, the concave radial head glides anteriorly on the capitulum along the capitulotrochlear groove. The reverse occurs in extension as the concave radial head glides posteriorly along the radial head in the capitulotrochlear groove. Forearm movements of rotation occur at this joint also and will be described in the next section on the proximal radioulnar joint. As with the humeroulnar joint, these motions usually occur in open kinetic chain, but with a closed kinetic chain movement such as pull-ups or pushups, the opposite can occur.

Proximal Radioulnar

The proximal or superior radioulnar joint is the primary joint that allows forearm rotation. There is at this joint a concave ulnar notch that articulates with the convex radial head. During the motions of pronation and supination, the radial head will rotate along the radius' long axis, creating a spinning at the superior radioulnar joint. This spinning will also occur at the radiohumeral joint described earlier. With the motion of pronation, the convex rim of the radial head will spin posteriorly in the concave ulnar notch (figure 8.6). With the motion of supination, the radial head will spin anteriorly in the concave radial notch.

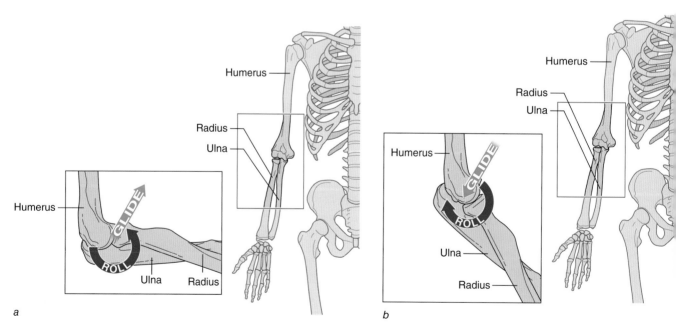

Figure 8.5 (a) Humeroulnar joint flexion. The trochlear ridge of the ulna glides anteriorly, superiorly, and laterally on the trochlear groove. (b) Humeroulnar joint extension. The trochlear ridge of the ulna glides posteriorly, inferiorly, and medially on the trochlear groove.

The proximal radioulnar joint is primarily responsible for forearm rotation motions of supination and pronation. These motions, however, are also intrinsically linked to the distal radioulnar joint. Therefore, a limitation of forearm rotation must require evaluation of passive movements of both the proximal and distal radioulnar joints.

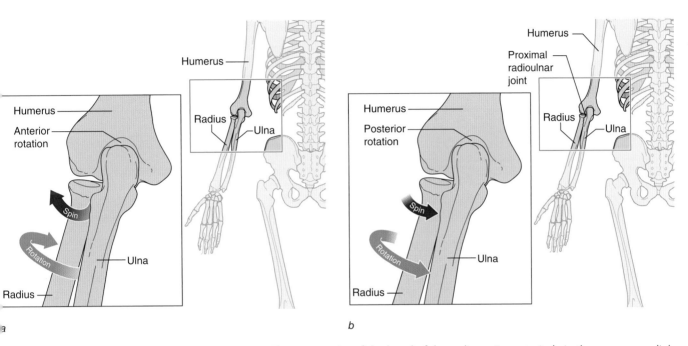

a

b

Figure 8.6 *(a)* Superior radioulnar joint pronation. The convex rim of the head of the radius spins anteriorly in the concave radial notch. *(b)* Superior radioulnar joint supination. The convex rim of the head of the radius spins posteriorly in the concave radial notch.

ELBOW JOINT ARTHROLOGY

Articular surfaces	Closed packed position	Resting position	Capsular pattern	ROM norms	End-feel
Humeroulnar					
Humerus: concave medial to lateral (abduction/adduction) Ulna: convex ventral to dorsal (flexion/extension)	Full extension and supination	70° flexion 10° supination	Flexion > extension	0°–150°	Flexion = soft tissue Extension = firm
Humeroradial					
Humerus: convex Radius: concave	90° elbow flexion, 5° supination	Full extension and supination	Flexion > extension Supination restricted only if condition is severe	0°–150°	Flexion = soft tissue Extension = firm
Proximal radioulnar					
Radius: convex Ulna: concave	5° supination Full extension	35° supination 70° flexion	Supination = pronation	Supination = 90° Pronation = 90°	Supination = firm Pronation = firm or bony
Distal radioulnar					
Radius: concave Ulna: convex	5° supination	10° supination	Supination = pronation	Supination = 90° Pronation = 90°	Supination = firm Pronation = firm or bony

Distraction, Loose Packed Position

VIDEO 8.1 **in the web study guide shows this technique.**

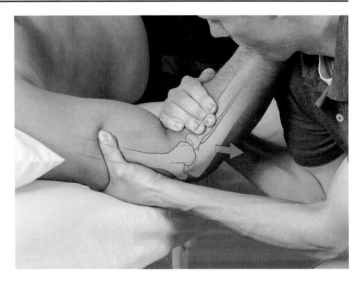

Client position: Supine, elbow flexed approximately 70° and supinated approximately 10°; distal forearm and hand resting on clinician's shoulder.

Clinician position: Sitting facing client's head; client's elbow in resting position if conservative technique is to be used.

Stabilization: Proximal hand grasps client's proximal humerus on the ventral side for stabilization.

Mobilization: Grasping the proximal ulna from the ventral side, clinician mobilizes the ulna away from the humeral joint surface at a 90° angle from the treatment plane, or at an angle 45° less flexion than the position of the ulnar shaft.

Goal of technique: To increase overall flexion and extension of the humeroulnar joint.

Notes: A clinician with small hands can grasp around the proximal ulna with fingers interlocked, allowing the weight of client's body to stabilize the humerus. Realize that this will also distract the humeroradial joint. This technique is general at best, not specific.

Medial Glide

VIDEO 8.2 **in the web study guide shows this technique.**

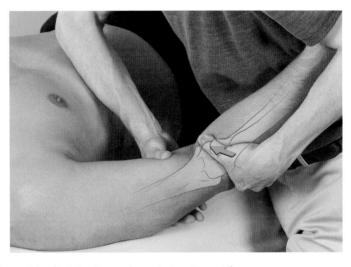

Client position: Supine, elbow flexed approximately 70°; forearm supinated 10° if conservative technique is to be used.

Clinician position: Standing facing client's head, holding the distal forearm between clinician's upper arm and trunk for stabilization.

Stabilization: Proximal hand contacts the distal humerus from the medial side, stabilizing the distal humerus.

Mobilization: Glide the proximal ulna in a medial direction indirectly through the radius with clinician's trunk assisting in guiding the motion.

Goal of technique: To increase overall humeroulnar flexion and extension.

Note: This is a great general mobilization to increase elbow flexion, extension, and abduction.

Lateral Glide

VIDEO 8.3 in the web study guide shows this technique.

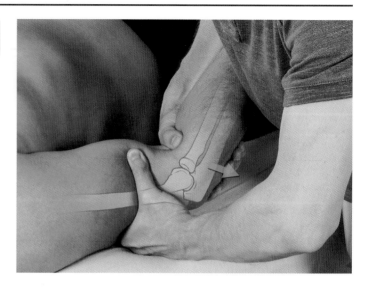

Client position: Supine, elbow flexed 70°; forearm supinated 10° if conservative technique is to be used.

Clinician position: Standing alongside client facing client's head, holding distal forearm between clinician's upper arm and trunk for stabilization.

Stabilization: Proximal hand will grip the distal humerus from the lateral side.

Mobilization: Distal hand will grip the proximal ulna from the medial side. While the stabilizing hand holds the humerus in place, the manipulating hand glides the proximal ulna in a lateral direction while clinician's trunk helps guide the motion.

Goal of technique: To increase overall humeroulnar flexion and extension.

Note: This is an excellent general mobilization for elbow flexion, extension, and adduction.

Medial Gap

Client position: Supine, elbow flexed 70°; forearm supinated 10° if conservative technique is to be used.

Clinician position: Standing alongside client's arm facing the humeroulnar joint with client's forearm between clinician's upper arm and trunk.

Stabilization: Distal hand supports forearm from the ulnar side and holds it against clinician's trunk.

Mobilization: Proximal hand moves elbow at the lateral joint line in a medial direction, creating a gapping at the joint line medially.

Goal of technique: To increase overall humeroulnar flexion and extension.

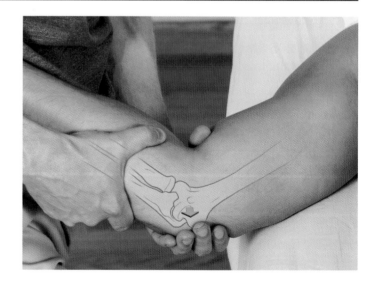

Notes: This is an alternate method that stabilizes the lateral distal humerus, while the manipulating hand grasps the proximal forearm ulnarly, moving this portion in a lateral direction, thus gapping the medial side of the joint.

Lateral Gap

Client position: Supine, elbow flexed 70°; forearm supinated 10° if conservative technique is to be used.

Clinician position: Standing at client's side, facing the humeroulnar joint with client's forearm between clinician's upper arm and trunk.

Stabilization: Clinician's distal hand holds client's forearm from the radial side against clinician's trunk.

Mobilization: Proximal hand grasps the medial side of elbow at the joint line, mobilizing the medial side of elbow in the lateral direction, thus creating a gap at the lateral joint line.

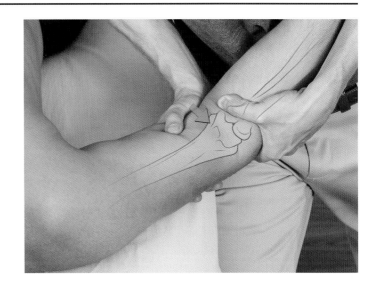

Goal of technique: To increase overall humeroulnar flexion and extension.

Notes: You can use an alternate technique similar to the medial gap alternate technique. Take care not to allow forearm pronation during this mobilization.

Distraction

▶ **VIDEO 8.4 in the web study guide shows this technique.**

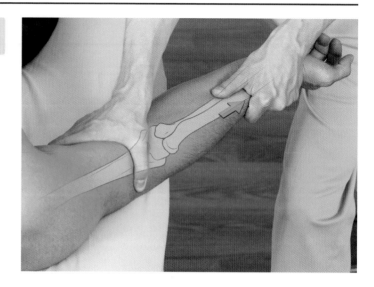

Client position: Supine, elbow in full extension; forearm in full supination if conservative technique is to be used.

Clinician position: Standing alongside client's elbow, facing cephalad.

Stabilization: Proximal hand grasps the distal humerus from the ventral side, while the distal hand grasps the distal radius.

Mobilization: The distal hand distracts the radius in a distal direction.

Goal of technique: To increase overall humeroradial mobility of flexion/extension and supination/pronation.

Notes: This is a great general technique to increase overall humeroradial motion. It is also helpful for reducing a proximal positional fault. The technique might also increase effect of distraction by ulnarly deviating the wrist, but note that you are now putting passive tension through wrist radial deviators and associated ligaments.

Compression

Client position: Supine, elbow positioned in 90° of elbow flexion, neutral rotation and wrist extension.

Clinician position: Standing alongside client, facing cephalad.

Stabilization: Clinician grasps the distal humerus from the dorsal side.

Mobilization: Distal hand moves the radius in a downward compressive direction indirectly through the wrist.

Goal of technique: To compress the humeroradial joint.

Notes: This technique is most often used to correct a distal positional fault of the radius. It might also increase the effect of compression by radially deviating the wrist, but note that you are now compressing through 2 joints.

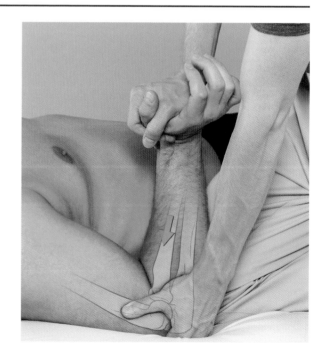

Radial Dorsal Glide

VIDEO 8.5 **in the web study guide shows this technique.**

Client position: Supine, elbow in full extension; forearm in supination if conservative technique is to be used.

Clinician position: Standing alongside client, facing cephalad.

Stabilization: Proximal hand grasps the distal humerus from the dorsal side.

Mobilization: Distal hand mobilizes the proximal radius in a dorsal direction on the humerus.

Goal of technique: To increase elbow extension and forearm pronation.

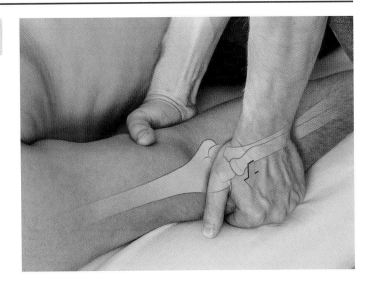

Radial Ventral Glide

VIDEO 8.6 **in the web study guide shows this technique.**

Client position: Supine, elbow in full extension; forearm in supination if conservative technique is to be used.

Clinician position: Sitting alongside client, facing client's side.

Stabilization: Proximal hand grasps the distal humerus from the ventral side.

Mobilization: Distal hand mobilizes the proximal radius in a ventral direction on the humerus.

Goal of technique: To increase elbow flexion and forearm supination.

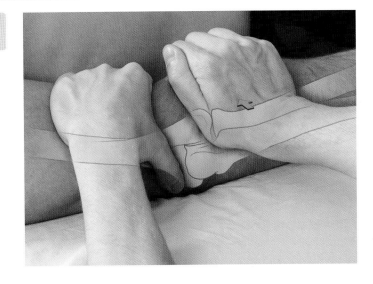

Dorsal Glide of the Radial Head

 VIDEO 8.7 in the web study guide shows this technique.

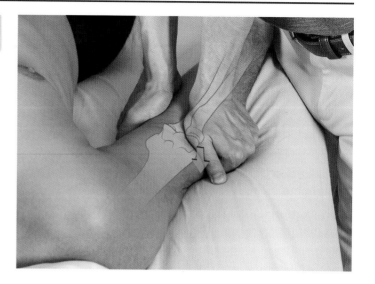

Client position: Sitting alongside treatment table, elbow on table, flexed 70°; forearm supinated 35° if conservative technique is to be used.

Clinician position: Standing, facing client on side to be mobilized.

Stabilization: Client's proximal ulna is grasped from the dorsal side.

Mobilization: The radial head is mobilized in a dorsal direction on the ulna.

Goal of technique: To gain motion of elbow extension and forearm pronation.

Ventral Glide of the Radial Head

 VIDEO 8.8 in the web study guide shows this technique.

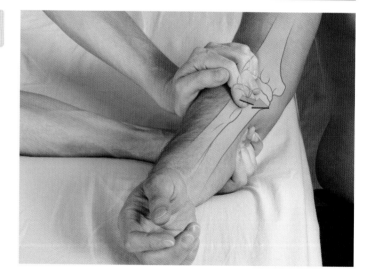

Client position: Sitting alongside treatment table, elbow on table, flexed 70° and supinated 35° if conservative technique is to be used.

Clinician position: Standing, facing client on side to be mobilized.

Stabilization: Client's proximal ulna is grasped from the ventral side.

Mobilization: The radial head is mobilized in a ventral direction on the ulna.

Goal of technique: To gain motion of elbow flexion and forearm supination.

Notes: This is an excellent technique to increase forearm supination. Take care to stabilize correctly because the arm will naturally want to fall into further pronation.

Dorsal Glide of the Radius

Client position: Sitting with forearm in 10° of supination if conservative technique is to be used.

Clinician position: Sitting alongside client, facing the distal radioulnar joint.

Stabilization: The distal ulna is grasped from the dorsal side.

Mobilization: The radius is mobilized in a dorsal direction on the distal ulna.

Goal of technique: To increase forearm supination.

Note: Remember that a dorsal glide of the radius is in effect imparting a ventral glide of the ulna.

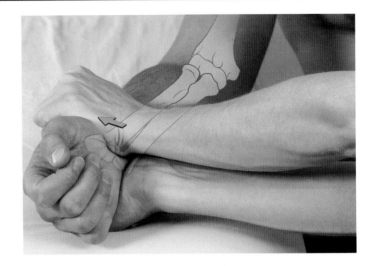

Ventral Glide of the Radius

Client position: Sitting with forearm in 10° of supination if conservative technique is to be used.

Clinician position: Sitting alongside client, facing the distal radioulnar joint.

Stabilization: The distal ulna is grasped from the ventral side.

Mobilization: The radius is mobilized in a ventral direction on the ulna.

Goal of technique: To increase forearm pronation.

Note: Remember that a ventral glide of the radius is in effect imparting a dorsal glide of the ulna.

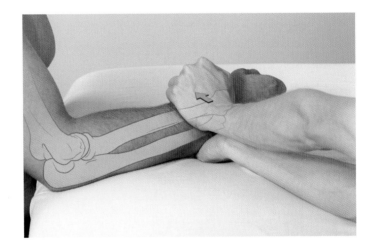

Go to the web study guide and complete the case study for this chapter. The case study discusses a 16-year-old baseball pitcher who injured his right elbow.

EVIDENCE FOR MANUAL THERAPY OF VARIOUS ELBOW JOINT PATHOLOGIES

Study	Clients	Intervention and comparison (if any)	Outcome(s)
Utilization of thrust and nonthrust mobilization for the elbow: Grade A			
Heiser R, O'Brien VH, Schwartz DA, 2013 (Level 2A)	Systematic review 22 studies 16 specific to elbow	Examine evidence describing joint mobilization for treatment of elbow, wrist, and hand conditions and offer practical clinical guidelines.	Moderate support for inclusion joint mobilizations for treatment of lateral epicondylalgia.

WRIST AND HAND

LEARNING OBJECTIVES

After completing this chapter, you will be able to do the following:

◆ Describe the bony and soft tissue anatomy of the wrist and hand complex

◆ Discuss the joint kinematics of the wrist and hand joint complex

◆ Describe appropriate positioning, movements, and intentions for the wrist and hand complex mobilization techniques

◆ Identify evidence supporting wrist and hand complex mobilization techniques

The wrist and hand make up a complex set of joints capable of numerous grips and grasps that allow the hand to perform countless functions. Stability of the wrist is essential for optimal function of the finger flexors and extensors to allow mobility of the hand. The hand is the distal link to the upper extremity kinetic chain and is dependent on strength and mobility of the shoulder, elbow, forearm, and wrist. Injuries to the wrist/hand complex can have devastating consequence for the function of the upper extremity. Common injuries include carpal tunnel syndrome, various fractures, and traumatic/nontraumatic tendon injuries.

Anatomy

The wrist and hand complex is comprised of multiple bones and synovial joints. The wrist complex consists of the distal radioulnar, radiocarpal, and midcarpal joints (figure 9.1). The hand contains the carpometacarpal, metacarpophalangeal, and interphalangeal joints. The thumb has unique anatomy and functions and will be described separately from the other 4 digits.

Distal Radioulnar Joint

The distal radioulnar articulation occurs between the convex ulnar head and concave ulnar notch of the radius. This joint is also united by an articulating disc, a part of the triangular fibrocartilage complex (TFCC) (figure 9.2). This disc binds the distal radius to the ulna and is the primary stabilizer of the distal radioulnar joint. This is a diarthrodial double pivot joint allowing the forearm rotation movement of supination and pronation. The function of the distal radioulnar joint is to transmit the load from the hand to the forearm. The stability of the distal radioulnar joint

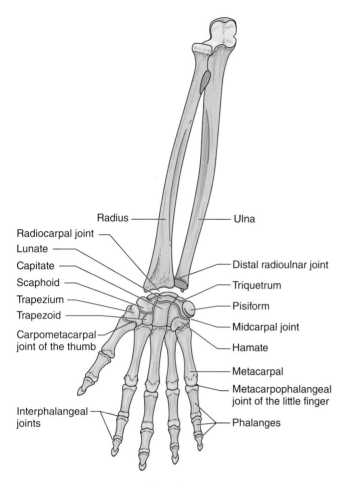

Figure 9.1 Wrist and hand joints.

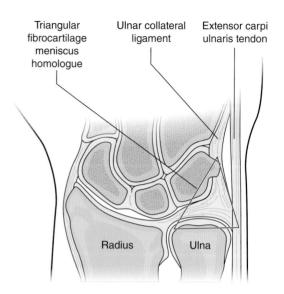

Figure 9.2 Triangular fibrocartilage complex (TFCC).

TFCC disc articulates with lunate and triquetrum (see figure 9.2). The ulna does not participate in the radiocarpal joint articulation besides serving as attachment site for the TFCC. The radiocarpal joint is a diarthrodial ellipsoid joint because its joint surfaces are ovoid and vary in length and curvature.

The wrist joint capsule encloses the distal radioulnar and the radiocarpal joints (the radius, ulna, triangular disc, and the proximal row of the carpals). The fibrous capsule is strong and loose and further reinforced by palmar and dorsal ligaments. The medial aspect of the wrist is stabilized by the ulnar collateral ligament, and the lateral aspect is stabilized by the radial collateral ligament (figure 9.3).

Midcarpal Joint

A complex articulation occurs between the proximal and distal rows of the carpal bones during wrist movements. The articulation is considered complex because each row has both a concave and a convex segment. The midcarpal joint is the S-shaped joint space separating the proximal and

is reinforced by the palmar and radial ligaments and the TFCC. The palmar radioulnar ligament runs from the anterior margin of the ulnar notch of the radius to the front of the head of the ulna. The dorsal radioulnar ligament runs from the posterior margin of the ulnar notch of the radius to the posterior head of the ulna.

Radiocarpal Joint

The radiocarpal joint is the articulation between the concave surface formed by the radial facets and TFCC disc with the convex surface of the following carpals: scaphoid, lunate, and triquetrum. The radius articulates with scaphoid and lunate. The

---

Clinical Tips

A Colles' fracture is a fracture of the distal radius with or without ulnar displacement. The most common mechanism of injury is a fall on an outstretched hand.

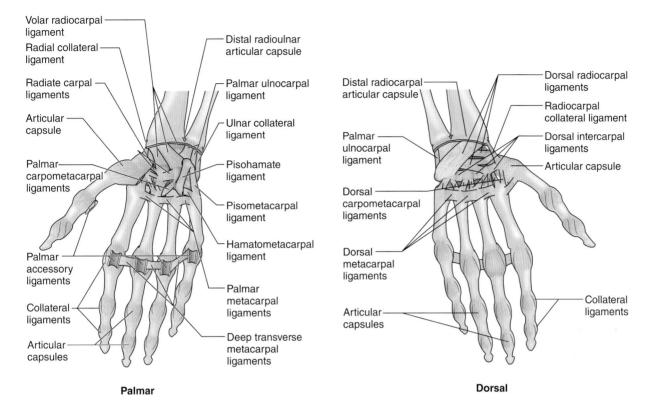

Palmar

Dorsal

Figure 9.3 Ligaments of the wrist and hand.

distal rows of the carpal bones. The articulation between the scaphoid, lunate, and triquetrum with the capitate and hamate forms a sellar joint on the medial side, whereas the articulation of the scaphoid with the trapezoid and trapezium forms another sellar joint on the lateral side. The midcarpal joint is classified as a diarthrodial condyloid joint that aids in wrist mobility (flexion, extension, radial deviation, and ulnar deviation). Some references classify this joint as a plane synovial joint.

The carpal bones and ligaments form a tunnel through which 9 flexor tendons and the median nerve pass. The floor of the carpal tunnel is covered by the palmar radiocarpal ligaments; the roof is formed by the flexor retinaculum (transverse carpal) ligament; the ulnar and radial boarders are formed by the trapezium and hook of the hamate respectively (figure 9.4). The median nerve is subject to compression within this tunnel.

Carpometacarpal Joints

The carpometacarpal joints are the articulations between the distal carpals and the base of the metacarpals; second metacarpal with the trapezium, trapezoid, and capitates; third metacarpal with the capitate; fourth metacarpal with the capitate and hamate; and fifth metacarpal with the hamate. These joints are diarthrodial condyloid joints. The mobility of the CMC joints is increased from the second to the fifth joint. The stability of these joints is provided by the palmar and dorsal carpometacarpal and intermetacarpal ligaments.

Clinical Tips

The carpal tunnel is the space within the wrist formed by the carpal bones and transverse carpal ligament. A common injury, carpal tunnel syndrome, involves compression of the median nerve within the tunnel. There is moderate evidence to show that joint mobilization is beneficial for individuals with carpal tunnel syndrome (Tal-Akabi and Rushton, 2000).

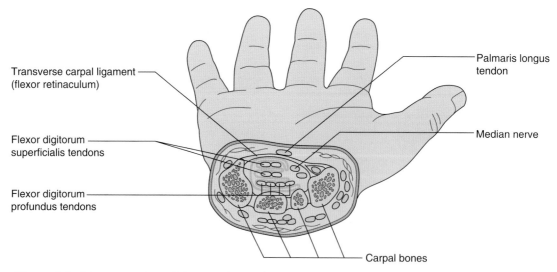

Figure 9.4 Transverse view of the carpal tunnel.

First Carpometacarpal Joint

This articulation occurs between the base of the first metacarpal and the distal surface of the trapezium. This is a diarthrodial sellar joint with reciprocal concavo-convex joint surfaces. The trapezium is concave in the anterior and posterior direction, and convex in the medial and lateral direction. The base of the first metacarpal is concave in the medial and lateral direction, and convex in the anterior and posterior direction.

Metacarpophalangeal Joints (MCPs)

The metacarpophalangeal joint is the articulation between the head of the metacarpal and its respective proximal phalange. These joints are diarthrodial condyloid joints. The head of the metacarpal has a biconvex shape that is broader anteriorly and narrower posteriorly; the phalanx is concave proximally.

Stability of the MCPs is provided by the medial and lateral collateral ligaments that run obliquely from the lateral aspect of the metacarpal head to the corresponding base of the phalanx on the side, facing palmarly (figure 9.5). The palmar aspect of the joint is covered by a dense fibrocartilaginous pad, the palmar ligament (volar plate), which prevents the hyperextension of the joints. The dorsal aspect of the joint is covered by the extensor aponeurosis (extensor expansion). The heads of the metacarpals are connected by deep transverse metacarpal ligaments.

Interphalangeal Joints

All 4 fingers have a proximal interphalangeal joint (PIP). The thumb has 1 interphalangeal joint. The PIP articulation occurs between the head of the proximal phalange and its respective middle phalange. The head of the proximal phalange of each digit has 2 separate convex shaped condyles (pulley shaped heads). The base of the middle

---

Clinical Tips

The most common location for osteoarthritis (OA) of the hand is the CMC joint of the thumb. Females are more prone to the development of OA in their fourth and fifth decades. OA to this joint is quite debilitating because of the frequent use of the joint with ADLs and fine motor tasks. Joint mobilization has been shown to be beneficial in decreasing pain in individuals with CMC OA (Villafañe, Cleland, and Fernández-de-las-peñas, 2013).

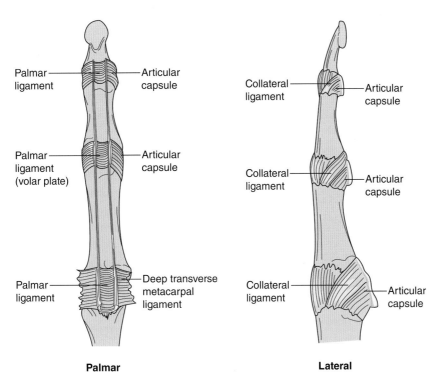

Figure 9.5 Ligaments of the MCP and IP joints.

phalanx of each digit has a concave base with 2 separate depressions. This is a hinged joint that allows flexion and extension motions. The distal interphalangeal joint (DIP) is similar to the PIP, with the exception that the distal joint is less stable and has more hyperextension.

Similar to the MCP joints, the interphalangeal joints are protected by collateral ligaments with oblique fibers. The palmar aspect of the joint contains a volar plate (palmar ligament), which is fixed proximally to the neck of its proximal phalanx and distally to the base of its distal phalanx (see figure 9.5). The volar plate also attaches to the flexor sheath and collateral ligament and prevents hyperextension of the joint.

Joint Kinematics

The joints of the wrist and hand are numerous, and joint motion traverses multiple planes. This joint complex is critical for function of the upper extremity. The clinician must have a good understanding of the intricacies of these joints in order to treat this area effectively.

Distal Radioulnar Joint

The distal radioulnar joint has 1 degree of freedom. The movements of supination and pronation occur simultaneously with movement at the proximal radioulnar joint in the transverse plane around the vertical axis. This vertical axis extends from the radial head to the ulnar head. With supination, the concave ulnar notch of the radius glides dorsally (posteriorly) on the ulnar head. The ulnar head moves proximally and medially in supination. Pronation is opposite, with the concave ulnar notch gliding volarly (anteriorly) on the ulnar head. The ulnar head moves distally and dorsally.

Radiocarpal Joint and Midcarpal Joint

The radiocarpal joint has 2 degrees of freedom, including wrist flexion and extension in the sagittal plane and radial and ulnar deviation in the frontal plane. Flexion and extension occurs in the sagittal plane around the medial/lateral axis that goes through the head of the capitate. Radial and ulnar deviation occurs in the frontal plane around the anterior/posterior axis that goes through the head of the capitate.

At the radiocarpal joint, the relatively convex proximal carpal row articulates with the concave radial facets and radioulnar disc. During flexion, the proximal carpal row (scaphoid and lunate) glides dorsally on the radius with the triquetrum gliding dorsally on the TFCC. About 35 degrees of flexion motion of the wrist occurs at the radiocarpal joint with the remaining motion occurring at the midcarpal joints. Flexion is also accompanied by slight ulnar deviation and supination.

Wrist extension involves the proximal carpal row (scaphoid and lunate) gliding volarly (anteriorly) on the concave surface of radius, whereas the triquetrum glides volarly on the radioulnar disc. Most of the extension motion occurs at the radiocarpal joint (45°), with the remainder occurring at the midcarpal joint. Extension is accompanied by slight radial deviation and pronation of the forearm (figure 9.6).

Ulnar deviation of the wrist is characterized by convex-on-concave movement at both radiocarpal and midcarpal joints. The proximal carpal row rolls ulnarly and glides radially at the radiocarpal joint. At the midcarpal joint, the capitate and hamate roll ulnarly and glide radially, and the trapezium and trapezoid glide palmarly. Radial deviation of the wrist is opposite of ulnar deviation. The proximal carpal row rolls radially and glides ulnarly at the

radiocarpal joint. At the midcarpal joint, the capitate and hamate roll radially and glide dorsally, and the trapezium and trapezoid glide dorsally.

Carpometacarpal Joints

The irregular shapes of the carpometacarpal joint surfaces don't allow for standard arthrokinematic description. The second and third digits have very little movement due to the interlocking articular surfaces. Movement at the fourth and fifth digits allows the ulnar border of the hand to fold toward the center of the hand, deepening the palmar concavity. Movement at the fourth and fifth metacarpal joint (MC) is referred to as ulnar mobility. The mobility in these medial joints allows a cupping motion of the hand.

First Carpometacarpal Joint

The CMC joint of the thumb has 2 degrees of freedom: flexion/extension and abduction/adduction. Flexion and extension occur in the frontal plane around the anterior/posterior axis through the trapezium. Abduction and adduction occur in the sagittal plane around the medial/lateral axis through the metacarpal. The motion of opposition is a combination of movements (including varying amounts of flexion, internal rotation, and adduction).

The CMC joint of the thumb consists of the concavo-convex base of the first metacarpal and

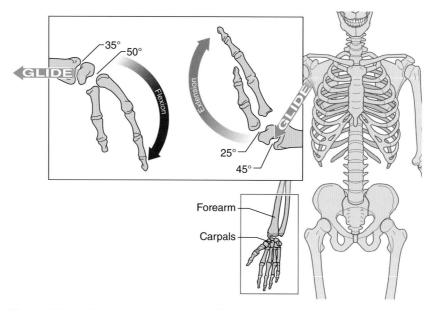

Figure 9.6 Radiocarpal and midcarpal flexion and extension.

the concavo-convex trapezium. The metacarpal is concave in the medial/lateral direction and convex in the anterior/posterior direction. Thumb flexion involves the concave surface of the metacarpal rolling and gliding in an ulnar (medial) direction. Extension is the reverse and consists of the metacarpal rolling and gliding in a radial (lateral) direction across the transverse diameter of the joint. The arthrokinematics of thumb abduction comprise a convex surface of the metacarpal rolling palmarly and gliding dorsally on the concave surface of the trapezium. During adduction, the metacarpal rolls dorsally and glides palmarly on the concave surface of the trapezium.

Metacarpophalangeal Joints

The metacarpal joints have 2 degrees of freedom: flexion/extension and abduction/adduction. Flexion and extension occur in the sagittal plane around a medial/lateral axis though the head of the metacarpal. Abduction and adduction occur in the frontal plane around an anterior/posterior axis through the head of the metacarpal.

The MCP articulation consists of a concave base of the phalanx and a convex metacarpal head. During flexion, the phalanx rolls and glides palmarly on the convex metacarpal. Extension involves the phalanx rolling and gliding dorsally on a convex metacarpal. During abduction and adduction, the proximal phalanx rolls and glides in the same direction of movement as the fingers (radially or ulnarly).

The thumb MCP is similar anatomically to digits 2 through 5. However, the orientation of movements is different. Flexion and extension occur primarily in the frontal plane around an anterior/posterior axis. Abduction and adduction occur primarily in the sagittal plane around the medial/lateral axis through the metacarpal. There is also a slight degree of axial rotation that occurs at the thumb. During flexion, the concave base of the proximal phalanx glides toward the palmar surface of the thumb. The opposite occurs during extension: the concave base of the proximal phalanx glides toward the dorsal surface. The arthrokinematics for the first MCP abduction involve the proximal phalanx rolling and gliding in the same direction as movement of the thumb. During adduction, the proximal phalanx rolls and glides in the same direction as the movement of the thumb.

Interphalangeal Joints

The PIP and DIP joints have 1 degree of freedom: flexion and extension. Flexion and extension occur in a sagittal plane around a medial/lateral axis. During flexion, the concave distal phalanx glides palmarly. Extension is achieved with the distal phalanx gliding dorsally.

WRIST AND HAND JOINT ARTHROLOGY

Articular surfaces	Closed packed position	Resting position	Capsular pattern	ROM norms	End-feel
Distal radioulnar joint					
Convex ulnar head and concave ulnar notch on the radius	5° supination	Midway between supination and pronation	Pain at extreme ranges of motion	Pronation: 80° Supination: 80°	Tissue stretch in both directions
Radiocarpal joint					
Convex proximal carpal row articulates with the concave radial facets and radioulnar disc	Extension with radial deviation	Resting position of hand with 10° of wrist flexion, slight ulnar deviation	Equal limitation of flexion and extension	Flexion: 80° Extension: 70° Ulnar deviation: 30° Radial deviation: 20°	Tissue stretch in all directions; extension and radial deviation can be hard
Midcarpal joints					
Proximal carpals (scaphoid, lunate, triquetrum, pisiform) and the distal carpals (trapezium, trapezoid, capitate, hamate)	Extension with ulnar deviation	Resting position of hand with 10° of wrist flexion, slight ulnar deviation	None defined	Combined movement with radiocarpal joint	Tissue stretch in all directions; extension and radial deviation can be hard
Carpometacarpal joints					
Concave base of metacarpals and respective carpals	Not defined	Functional position of the hand	Equal limitation in all planes	None defined	Not defined
First CMC of the thumb					
Trapezium and first metacarpal; MC is concave in the medial/lateral direction and is convex in the anterior/posterior direction	Full thumb opposition	Midabduction and midflexion	Abduction limited greatest followed by extension	Flexion: 15° Extension: 80° Abduction: 70°	Tissue stretch in all directions; flexion and opposition may be soft
Metacarpophalangeal joints					
Convex distal metacarpal and the concave proximal phalanx	Full flexion	Slight flexion	Equal restrictions in flexion and extension	Flexion: 90° Extension: 30° Abduction: 80° Thumb flexion: 50°	Tissue stretch in all directions; extension is hard
Interphalangeal joints					
Convex proximal phalanx and the concave distal phalanx	Full extension	Slight flexion	Equal restrictions in flexion and extension	2–5 PIP flexion: 100° 2–5 DIP flexion: 90° Thumb DIP flexion: 80°	Flexion can be hard, firm, or soft. Extension: tissue stretch

Ventral (Palmar) Glide

Client position: Seated with forearm in neutral rotation and resting on treatment table.

Clinician position: Standing or sitting, facing the dorsum of client's distal radioulnar joint.

Stabilization: The stabilizing hand grasps the distal ulna from the dorsal side.

Mobilization: The mobilizing hand grips the distal radius from the dorsal side. While the stabilizing hand holds the ulna in position, the mobilizing hand glides the distal radius forward to elicit a ventral glide.

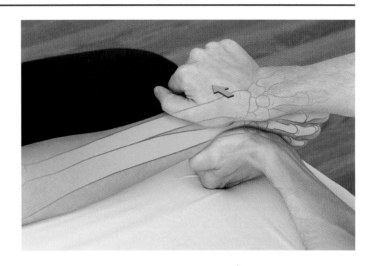

Goal of technique: To increase forearm pronation.

Note: Remember that a ventral glide of the radius is in effect imparting a dorsal glide of the ulna.

Dorsal Glide

Client position: Seated with forearm in neutral rotation and resting on treatment table.

Clinician position: Standing or sitting, facing the volar surface of client's distal radioulnar joint.

Stabilization: Clinician's stabilizing hand grasps the distal ulna from the dorsal side.

Mobilization: The mobilizing hand grips the distal radius from the ventral side. While the stabilizing hand holds the ulna in position, the mobilizing hand glides the distal radius back to elicit a dorsal glide.

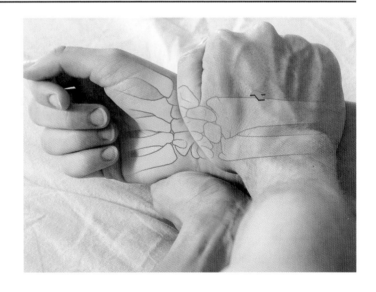

Goal of technique: To increase forearm supination.

Note: A dorsal glide of the radius is in effect imparting a volar glide of the ulna.

Distraction

Client position: Sitting with ventral forearm on treatment table and hand off edge of table. Keep radiocarpal (RC) and ulnocarpal (UC) joints in resting open packed position.

Clinician position: Standing facing the radiocarpal and ulnocarpal joints to be treated.

Stabilization: Clinician's proximal hand stabilizes at the distal radius and ulna from the dorsal aspect of client's forearm. This hand stabilizes client's distal forearm against treatment table.

Mobilization: Clinician's mobilizing hand grabs the proximal row of carpals from the dorsal side. The mobilizing hand pulls the proximal carpal row from the radius and ulna to elicit a distraction at this joint.

Goal of technique: To increase general mobility and inhibit pain.

Note: This technique may add varying degrees of flexion and extension and ulnar or radial deviation.

Dorsal Glide

 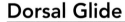 **VIDEO 9.1 in the web study guide shows this technique.**

Client position: Sitting, with either ulnar aspect or dorsal forearm on treatment table and hand off edge of table. Keep RC and UC joints in resting open packed position.

Clinician position: Standing facing the radiocarpal and ulnocarpal joints to be treated.

Stabilization: Clinician's proximal hand stabilizes at the distal radius and ulna from the dorsal aspect of client's forearm. This hand stabilizes the client's distal forearm against the treatment table.

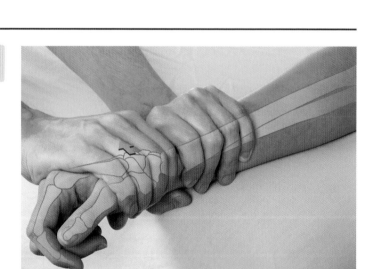

Mobilization: Clinician's mobilizing hand grabs the proximal row of carpals from the dorsal side. The mobilizing hand pulls the proximal carpal row toward clinician to elicit a dorsal glide.

Goal of technique: To increase general mobility and wrist flexion.

Note: The client might need to rotate the shoulder and body slightly to keep the wrist in neutral position.

Ventral Glide

Client position: Sitting, with either ulnar aspect or dorsal forearm on treatment table and hand off edge of table. Keep RC and UC joints in resting open packed position.

Clinician position: Standing facing the radiocarpal and ulnocarpal joints to be treated.

Stabilization: Clinician's proximal hand stabilizes at the distal radius and ulna from the dorsal aspect of client's forearm. This hand stabilizes client's distal forearm against treatment table.

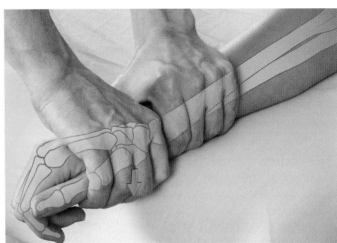

Mobilization: Clinician's mobilizing hand grabs the proximal row of carpals from the dorsal side. The mobilizing hand glides the proximal carpal row ventral.

Goal of technique: To increase general mobility and wrist extension.

Note: The client might need to rotate the shoulder and body slightly to keep the wrist in neutral position.

Radial Glide

Client position: Sitting with ventral forearm on treatment table and hand off edge of table. Keep RC and UC joints in resting open packed position.

Clinician position: Sitting facing the radiocarpal and ulnocarpal joints to be treated.

Stabilization: Clinician's proximal hand stabilizes at the distal radius and ulna from the dorsal aspect of client's forearm. This hand stabilizes client's distal forearm against treatment table.

Mobilization: Clinician's mobilizing hand grabs the proximal row of carpals from the dorsal side. The mobilizing hand glides the proximal carpal row toward the radius to elicit a radial glide. There is a better biomechanical advantage if clinician mobilizes away from his or her body rather than toward his or her body.

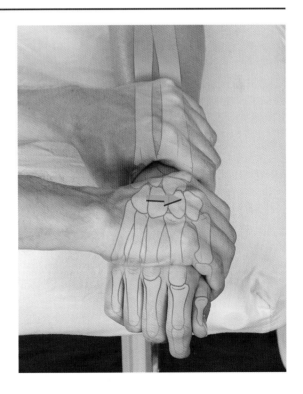

Goal of technique: To increase ulnar deviation.

Notes: The client might need to rotate the shoulder and body slightly to keep the wrist in neutral position. This technique is also good for articular nourishment to wrist structures.

Ulnar Glide

Client position: Sitting, with either ulnar aspect or dorsal forearm on treatment table and hand off edge of table. Keep RC and UC joints in resting open packed position.

Clinician position: Standing facing the radiocarpal and ulnocarpal joints to be treated.

Stabilization: Clinician's proximal hand stabilizes at the distal radius and ulna from the ventral aspect of client's forearm. This hand stabilizes client's distal forearm against treatment table.

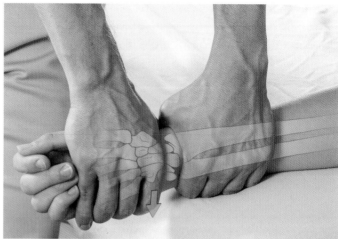

Mobilization: Clinician's mobilizing hand grabs the proximal row of carpals from the radial side. The mobilizing hand glides the proximal carpal row toward the ulna to elicit an ulnar glide.

Goal of technique: To increase radial deviation.

Note: The client might need to rotate the shoulder and body slightly to keep the wrist in neutral position.

Mobilizations for Scaphoid, Lunate, and Triquetrum for Restricted Extension

VIDEO 9.2 in the web study guide shows this technique.

Client position: Sitting with ventral aspect of forearm on treatment table. Keep RC and UC joints in resting open packed position.

Clinician position: Standing facing the radiocarpal and ulnocarpal joints to be treated.

Stabilization: Clinician's proximal hand stabilizes at the distal radius and ulna with thumb on the dorsal surface and remaining digits on the ventral surface. Additional stabilization can be used by clinician holding client's hand against clinician's trunk.

Mobilization: Clinician's mobilizing hand grips the given proximal carpal with thumb on the dorsal surface and index finger on the volar surface. The mobilizing hand mobilizes the given proximal carpal bone downward to elicit a volar glide. (a) The scaphoid is mobilized on the radius, (b) the lunate on the radius, and (c) the triquetrum on the triangular fibrocartilage disc.

Goal of technique: To increase wrist extension.

Notes: The client might need to rotate the shoulder and body slightly to keep the wrist in neutral position. This technique is also good for articular nourishment to wrist structures.

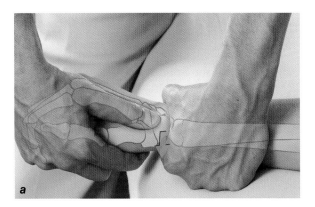

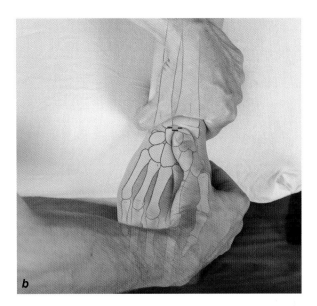

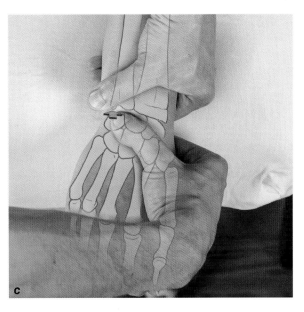

Mobilizations for Scaphoid, Lunate, and Triquetrum for Restricted Flexion

VIDEO 9.2 in the web study guide shows this technique.

Client position: Sitting with ventral aspect of forearm on treatment table. Keep RC and UC joints in resting open packed position.

Clinician position: Standing facing the radiocarpal and ulnocarpal joints to be treated.

Stabilization: Clinician's proximal hand stabilizes at the distal radius and ulna with thumb on dorsal surface and remaining digits on ventral surface. Additional stabilization can be used by clinician holding client's hand against clinician's trunk.

Mobilization: Clinician's mobilizing hand grips the given proximal carpal with thumb on dorsal surface and index finger on volar surface. The mobilizing hand mobilizes the given proximal carpal bone upward to elicit a dorsal glide. *(a)* The scaphoid is mobilized on the radius, *(b)* the lunate on the radius, and *(c)* the triquetrum on the disc.

Goals of technique: To increase wrist flexion; to reduce a volar positional fault of the lunate when the lunate is being mobilized dorsally on the ulna.

Note: The client might need to rotate the shoulder and body slightly to keep the wrist in neutral position.

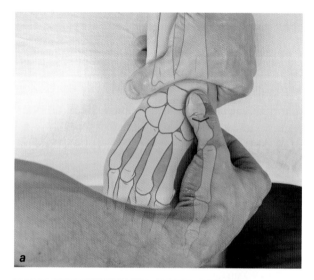

a

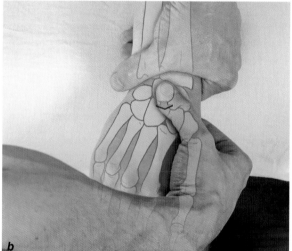

b

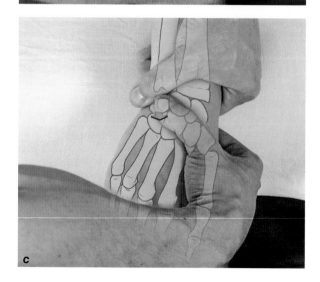

c

Distraction

VIDEO 9.3 **in the web study guide shows this technique.**

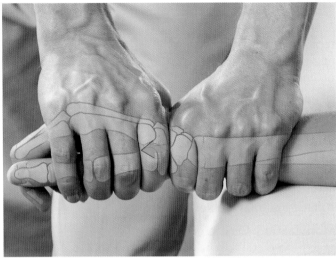

Client position: Sitting with ventral forearm on treatment table and hand off edge of table. Keep midcarpal joint in resting open packed position.

Clinician position: Standing facing the midcarpal joint on the treating arm.

Stabilization: Clinician's proximal hand stabilizes the proximal carpal row from the dorsal aspect of client's wrist. This hand also stabilizes client's distal forearm against treatment table.

Mobilization: Clinician's mobilizing hand grabs the distal row of carpals from the dorsal side. The mobilizing hand distracts the distal carpal row from the proximal carpal row.

Goal of technique: To increase general mobility and inhibit pain.

Note: The clinician might choose to add varying degrees of flexion and extension and ulnar or radial deviation.

Dorsal Glide

Client position: Sitting, with either ulnar aspect or dorsal forearm on treatment table and hand off edge of table. Keep midcarpal joint in resting open packed position.

Clinician position: Standing facing the midcarpal joint on the treating arm.

Stabilization: Clinician's proximal hand stabilizes the proximal carpal row from the dorsal aspect of client's wrist. This hand also stabilizes client's distal forearm against treatment table.

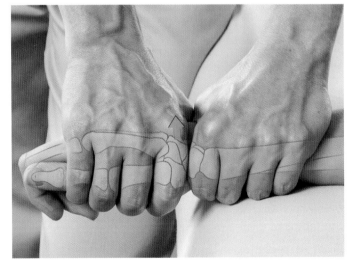

Mobilization: Clinician's mobilizing hand grabs the distal row of carpals from the dorsal side. The mobilizing hand pulls the distal carpal row back to elicit a dorsal glide.

Goal of technique: To increase wrist flexion.

Note: The client might need to rotate the shoulder and body slightly to keep the wrist in neutral position.

Ventral Glide

Client position: Sitting, with either ulnar aspect or ventral forearm on treatment table and hand off edge of table. Keep midcarpal joint in resting open packed position.

Clinician position: Standing facing the midcarpal joint on the treating arm.

Stabilization: Clinician's proximal hand stabilizes the proximal carpal row from the dorsal aspect of client's wrist. This hand also stabilizes client's distal forearm against treatment table.

Mobilization: Clinician's mobilizing hand grabs the distal row of carpals from the dorsal side. The mobilizing hand glides the distal carpal row downward in a ventral (volar) direction.

Goal of technique: To increase extension.

Note: The client might need to rotate the shoulder and body slightly to keep the wrist in neutral position.

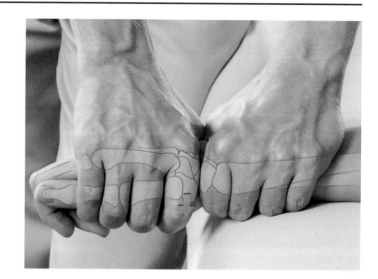

Radial Glide

Client position: Sitting, with either ulnar aspect or ventral forearm on treatment table and hand off edge of table. Keep midcarpal joint in resting open packed position.

Clinician position: Standing or sitting facing the midcarpal joint on the treating arm.

Stabilization: Clinician's proximal hand stabilizes the proximal carpal row from the dorsal aspect of client's wrist. This hand also stabilizes client's distal forearm against treatment table.

Mobilization: Clinician's mobilizing hand grabs the distal row of carpals from the ulnar side. The mobilizing hand glides the distal carpal row toward the radius to elicit a radial glide.

Goal of technique: To increase ulnar deviation at the wrist.

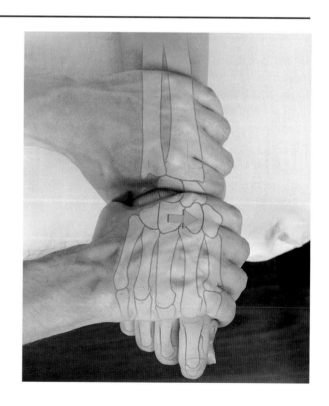

Ulnar Glide

Client position: Sitting with ulnar aspect of forearm on treatment table and hand off edge of table. Keep midcarpal joint in resting open packed position.

Clinician position: Standing facing the midcarpal joint on the treating arm.

Stabilization: Clinician's proximal hand stabilizes the proximal carpal row from the volar aspect of client's wrist. This hand also stabilizes client's distal forearm against treatment table.

Mobilization: Clinician's mobilizing hand grabs the distal row of carpals from the radial side. The mobilizing hand glides the distal carpal row toward the ulna to elicit an ulnar glide.

Goal of technique: To increase radial deviation at the wrist.

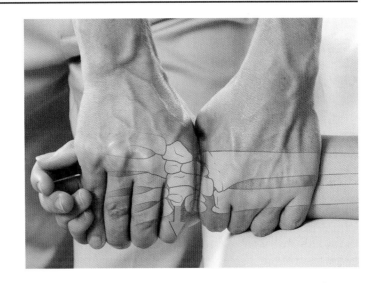

Midcarpal Extension Mobilization

Client position: Sitting with ventral aspect of forearm on treatment table. Keep midcarpal joints in resting open packed position.

Clinician position: Sitting facing the midcarpal joint on the treating arm.

Stabilization: The stabilizing hand grasps the proximal carpal bone with thumb on dorsal aspect and index finger on volar surface. Additional stabilization can be achieved by holding client's hand against clinician's trunk.

Mobilization: The mobilizing hand grips the distal carpal bone with thumb on dorsal surface and index finger on volar surface. The stabilizing hand holds the proximal carpal bone in place, while the mobilizing hand glides the *(a)* trapezium and trapezoid in a dorsal direction on the scaphoid, *(b)* the capitate in a volar direction on the scaphoid, *(c)* the capitate in a volar direction on the lunate, and *(d)* the hamate in a volar direction on the triquetrum.

Goal of technique: To increase wrist extension.

Note: This technique is good for articular nourishment to wrist structures.

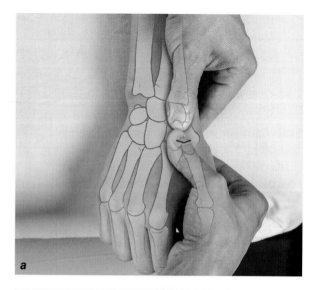

a

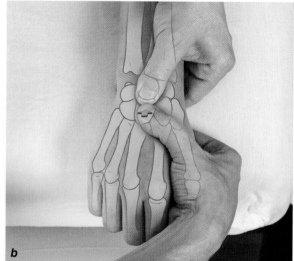

b

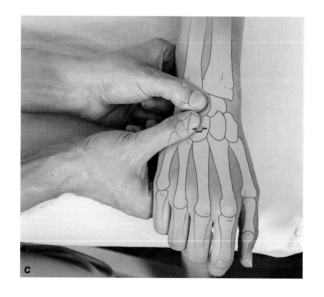

c

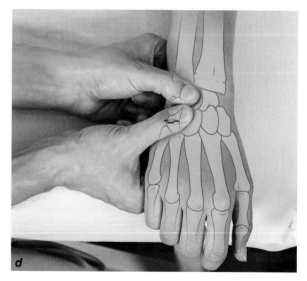

d

Midcarpal Flexion Mobilization

Client position: Sitting with ventral aspect of forearm on treatment table. Keep RC and UC joints in resting open packed position.

Clinician position: Sitting facing the midcarpal joint on the treating arm.

Stabilization: Clinician's proximal hand stabilizes at the distal radius and ulna with thumb on the dorsal surface and index finger on the ventral surface. Additional stabilization can be achieved by clinician holding client's hand against clinician's trunk.

Mobilization: The mobilizing hand grips the distal carpal bone with thumb on the dorsal surface and index finger on the volar surface. The stabilizing hand holds the proximal carpal bone in place, while the mobilizing hand glides the *(a)* trapezium and trapezoid in a volar direction on the scaphoid, *(b)* the capitate in a dorsal direction on the scaphoid, *(c)* the capitate in a dorsal direction on the lunate, and *(d)* the hamate in a dorsal direction on the triquetrum.

Goal of technique: To increase wrist flexion.

Note: This technique is good for articular nourishment to wrist structures.

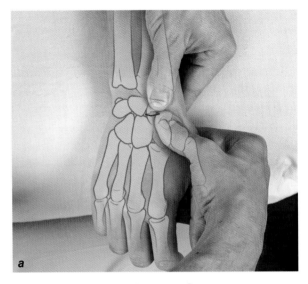

a

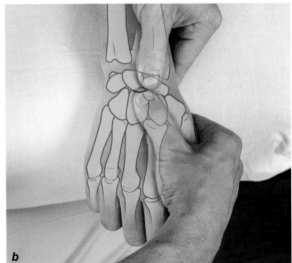

b

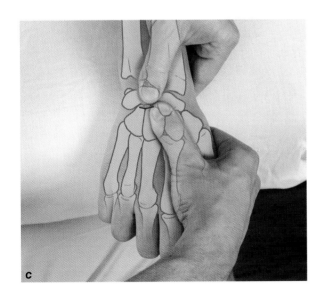

c

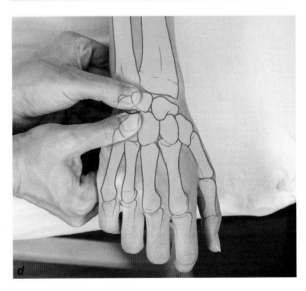

d

Intercarpal Mobilization

Client position: Sitting with ventral aspect of forearm on the treatment table. Keep RC and UC joints in resting open packed position.

Clinician position: Sitting facing the midcarpal joint on the treating arm.

Stabilization: Stabilizing hand grasps the proximal carpal bone with thumb on the dorsal aspect and index finger on the volar surface. Additional stabilization can be achieved by holding the client's hand against clinician's trunk.

Mobilization: The mobilizing hand grips 1 carpal bone with thumb on dorsal surface and index finger on volar surface. The stabilizing hand holds the carpal bone in place, while the mobilizing hand glides (a) the trapezoid in a dorsal direction on the capitate, (b) the trapezoid in a volar direction on the capitate, (c) the hamate in a dorsal direction on the capitate, and (d) the hamate in a volar direction on the capitate.

Goal of technique: To increase joint play among the distal row of carpals.

Note: This technique is good for articular nourishment to wrist structures.

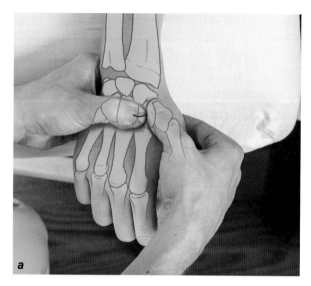

a

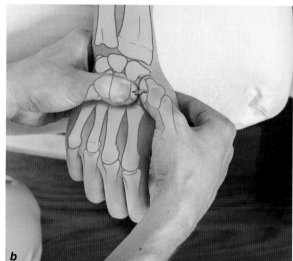

b

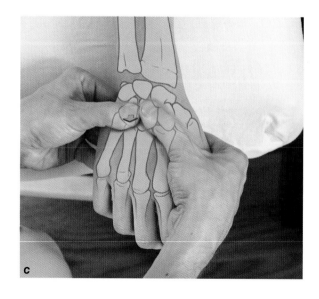

c

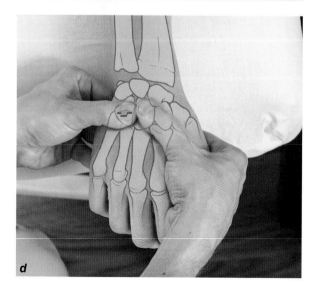

d

CMC Distraction

Client position: Sitting with forearm on treatment table, palm down.

Clinician position: Sitting facing the CMC to be treated.

Stabilization: Clinician's proximal hand stabilizes carpal bone of joint to be mobilized by placing thumb on dorsal surface and index finger on volar surface. Additional stabilization can be achieved by holding client's hand against clinician's trunk.

Mobilization: Clinician's mobilizing hand grips the base of the metacarpal of the joint being distracted with thumb on dorsal surface and index finger on volar surface. The mobilizing hand mobilizes the second metacarpal distal on the trapezoid, the third metacarpal distal on the capitate, the fourth metacarpal distal on the hamate, and the fifth metacarpal distal on the hamate.

Goal of technique: To promote joint play in digits 2 through 5.

Note: Movements in these joints are minimal, especially in the stable column of rays 2 and 3.

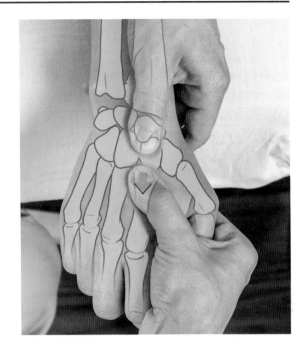

CMC Dorsal Glide

> **VIDEO 9.4 in the web study guide shows this technique.**

Client position: Sitting with forearm on treatment table, palm down.

Clinician position: Sitting facing the CMC to be treated.

Stabilization: Clinician's proximal hand stabilizes the carpal bone of the joint to be mobilized by placing thumb on the dorsal surface and index finger on the volar surface. Additional stabilization can be achieved by holding the client's hand against clinician's trunk.

Mobilization: Clinician's mobilizing hand grips the base of the metacarpal of the joint being mobilized with thumb on dorsal surface and index finger on volar surface. The mobilizing hand mobilizes the metacarpal upward to elicit a dorsal glide.

Goal of technique: To promote wrist/finger extension.

Note: Movements in these joints are minimal, especially in the stable column of rays 2 and 3.

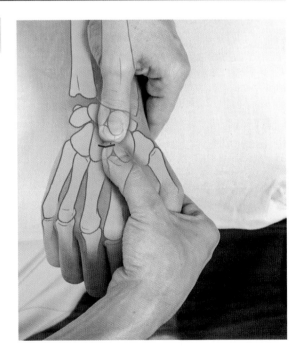

CMC Ventral Glide

 VIDEO 9.5 in the web study guide shows this technique.

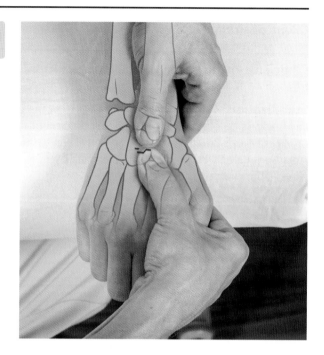

Client position: Sitting with forearm on treatment table, palm down.

Clinician position: Sitting facing the CMC to be treated.

Stabilization: Clinician's proximal hand stabilizes the carpal bone of the joint to be mobilized by placing thumb on the dorsal surface and index finger on the volar surface. Additional stabilization can be achieved by holding client's hand against clinician's trunk.

Mobilization: Clinician's mobilizing hand grips base of the metacarpal of joint being mobilized with thumb on dorsal surface and index finger on volar surface. The mobilizing hand mobilizes the metacarpal downward to elicit a volar glide.

Goal of technique: To increase wrist/finger flexion.

Note: Movements in these joints are minimal, especially in the stable column of rays 2 and 3.

Intermetacarpal Dorsal Glide

Client position: Sitting with forearm on treatment table, palm down.

Clinician position: Sitting facing the metacarpals to be treated.

Stabilization: Clinician's proximal hand stabilizes the midshaft of the metacarpal with thumb on dorsal surface and index finger on volar surface. Additional stabilization can be achieved by holding client's hand against clinician's trunk.

Mobilization: Clinician's mobilizing hand grips the midshaft of the other metacarpal with thumb on the dorsal surface and index finger on the volar surface. The stabilizing hand holds the metacarpal in position, while the mobilizing hand glides the second metacarpal in a dorsal direction on the third metacarpal, the fourth in a dorsal direction on the third, and the firth metacarpal in the dorsal direction on the fourth.

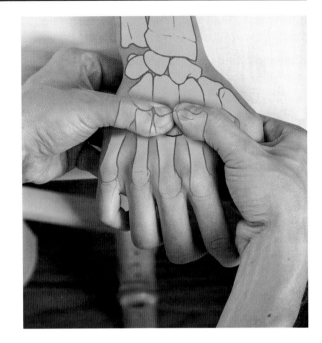

Goals of technique: To facilitate joint play in metacarpal articulations; to increase ROM for arch of the hand.

Note: This is also a good technique for nourishment of the joint's articular cartilage.

Intermetacarpal Ventral Glide

Client position: Sitting with forearm on treatment table, palm down.

Clinician position: Sitting facing the metacarpals to be treated.

Stabilization: Clinician's proximal hand stabilizes the midshaft of the first metacarpal with thumb on the dorsal surface and index finger on the volar surface. Additional stabilization can be achieved by holding client's hand against clinician's trunk.

Mobilization: Clinician's mobilizing hand grips the midshaft of the other metacarpal with thumb on the dorsal surface and index finger on the volar surface. The stabilizing hand holds the metacarpal in position, while the mobilizing hand glides the second metacarpal in a volar direction on the third metacarpal, the fourth in a volar direction on the third, and the firth metacarpal in the volar direction on the fourth.

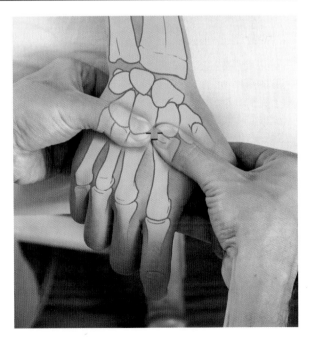

Goals of technique: To facilitate joint play in metacarpal articulations; to increase ROM for arch of the hand.

Note: This is also a good technique for nourishment of the joint's articular cartilage.

MCP Distraction

Client position: Sitting with forearm in neutral position.

Clinician position: Sitting facing the metacarpals to be treated.

Stabilization: Clinician's proximal hand stabilizes the head of the metacarpal of the joint to be mobilized with thumb on the dorsal surface and index finger on the volar surface. Additional stabilization can be achieved by holding client's hand against clinician's trunk.

Mobilization: Clinician's mobilizing hand grips the proximal end of the proximal phalanx being mobilized with thumb on the dorsal surface and index finger on the volar surface. The stabilizing hand holds the metacarpal in position, while the mobilizing hand glides the proximal phalanx distal to impart a distraction to the MCP joint.

Goals of technique: To facilitate joint play in metacarpal articulations; to increase ROM for arch of the hand.

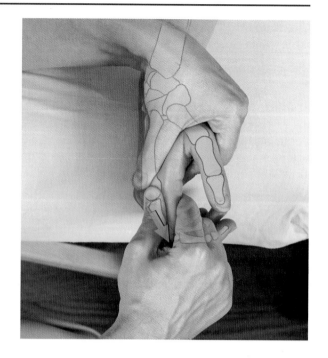

MCP Dorsal Glide

Client position: Sitting with forearm in neutral position.

Clinician position: Sitting facing the metacarpals to be treated.

Stabilization: Clinician's proximal hand stabilizes the head of the metacarpal of the joint to be mobilized with thumb on the dorsal surface and index finger on the volar surface. Additional stabilization can be achieved by holding client's hand against clinician's trunk.

Mobilization: Clinician's mobilizing hand grips the proximal end of the proximal phalanx being mobilized with thumb on the dorsal surface and index finger on the volar surface. The stabilizing hand holds the metacarpal in position, while the mobilizing hand glides the proximal phalanx in a posterior direction to elicit a dorsal glide.

Goals of technique: To facilitate joint play in metacarpal articulations; to increase ROM into MCP extension.

Note: This is also a good technique for nourishment of the joint's articular cartilage.

MCP Ventral Glide

Client position: Sitting with forearm in neutral position.

Clinician position: Standing or sitting facing the metacarpals to be treated.

Stabilization: Clinician's proximal hand stabilizes the head of the metacarpal of the joint to be mobilized with thumb on the dorsal surface and index finger on the volar surface. Additional stabilization can be achieved by holding client's hand against clinician's trunk.

Mobilization: Clinician's mobilizing hand grips the proximal end of the proximal phalanx being mobilized with thumb on the dorsal surface and index finger on the volar surface. The stabilizing hand holds the metacarpal in position, while the mobilizing hand glides the proximal phalanx in an anterior direction to elicit a ventral glide.

Goals of technique: To facilitate joint play in metacarpal articulations; to increase ROM into MCP flexion.

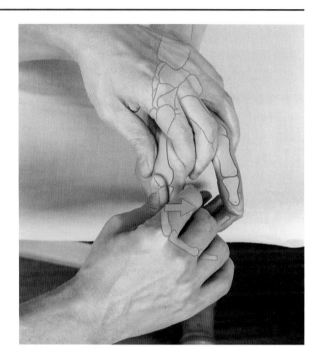

MCP Radial Glide

Client position: Sitting with palm facing down.

Clinician position: Standing or sitting facing the metacarpals to be treated.

Stabilization: Clinician's proximal hand stabilizes the head of the metacarpal of the joint to be mobilized with thumb on the ulnar surface and index finger on the radial surface. Additional stabilization can be achieved by holding client's hand against clinician's trunk.

Mobilization: Clinician's mobilizing hand grips the proximal end of the proximal phalanx being mobilized with thumb on the dorsal surface and index finger on the volar surface. The stabilizing hand holds the metacarpal in position, while the mobilizing hand glides the proximal phalanx in a radial direction to elicit a radial glide.

Goals of technique: To facilitate joint play in metacarpal articulations; to increase ROM for MCP abduction of digits 1 and 2, radial abduction of digit 3, and adduction of digits 4 and 5.

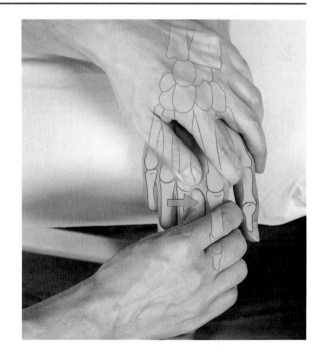

Note: This is also a good technique for nourishment of the joint's articular cartilage.

MCP Ulnar Glide

Client position: Sitting with palm facing down.

Clinician position: Standing or sitting facing the metacarpals to be treated.

Stabilization: Clinician's proximal hand stabilizes the head of the metacarpal of the joint to be mobilized with thumb on the ulnar surface and index finger on the radial surface. Additional stabilization can be achieved by holding client's hand against clinician's trunk.

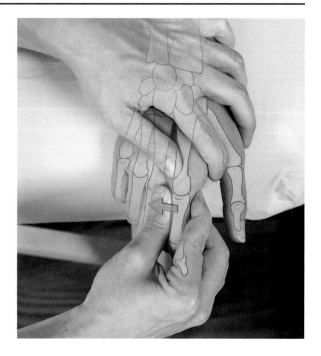

Mobilization: Clinician's mobilizing hand grips the proximal end of the proximal phalanx being mobilized with thumb on the dorsal surface and index finger on the volar surface. The stabilizing hand holds the metacarpal in position, while the mobilizing hand glides the proximal phalanx in an ulnar direction to elicit an ulnar glide.

Goals of technique: To facilitate joint play in metacarpal articulations; to increase ROM for MCP adduction of digits 1 and 2, ulnar abduction of digit 3, and abduction of digits 4 and 5.

Note: This is also a good technique for nourishment of the joint's articular cartilage.

IP Distraction

VIDEO 9.6 **in the web study guide shows this technique.**

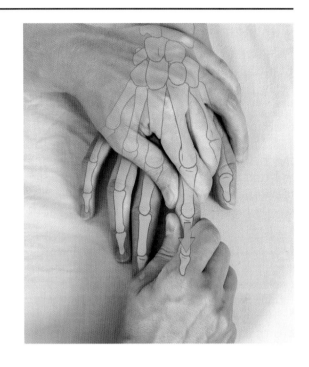

Client position: Sitting with palm facing down.

Clinician position: Standing or sitting facing the interphalangeal joint to be treated.

Stabilization: Clinician's proximal hand stabilizes the more proximal phalanx of the joint to be mobilized with thumb on the dorsal surface and index finger on the volar surface. Additional stabilization can be achieved by holding client's hand against clinician's trunk.

Mobilization: Clinician's mobilizing hand grips the proximal end of the more distal phalanx of the joint to be mobilized with thumb on the dorsal surface and index finger on the volar surface. The stabilizing hand holds the proximal phalanx in position while the mobilizing hand moves the distal phalanx distally to impart a distraction to the interphalangeal joint.

Goal of technique: To facilitate joint play in interphalangeal joints.

Note: This is also a good technique for nourishment of the joint's articular cartilage.

IP Dorsal Glide

VIDEO 9.7 **in the web study guide shows this technique.**

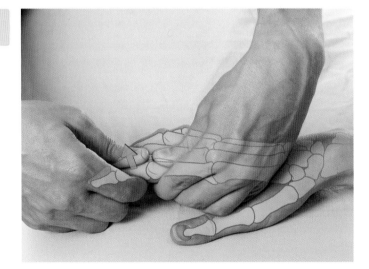

Client position: Sitting with palm facing down.

Clinician position: Standing or sitting facing the interphalangeal joint to be treated.

Stabilization: Clinician's proximal hand stabilizes the more proximal phalanx of the joint to be mobilized with thumb on the dorsal surface and index finger on the volar surface. Additional stabilization can be achieved by holding client's hand against clinician's trunk.

Mobilization: Clinician's mobilizing hand grips the proximal end of the more distal phalanx of the joint to be mobilized with thumb on the dorsal surface and index finger on the volar surface. The stabilizing hand holds the proximal phalanx in position while the mobilizing hand moves the distal phalanx in a posterior direction to elicit a dorsal glide.

Goals of technique: To facilitate joint play in interphalangeal joints and aid in interphalangeal joint extension.

Note: This is also a good technique for nourishment of the joint's articular cartilage.

IP Ventral Glide

Client position: Sitting with palm facing down.

Clinician position: Standing or sitting facing the interphalangeal joint to be treated.

Stabilization: Clinician's proximal hand stabilizes the more proximal phalanx of the joint to be mobilized with thumb on the dorsal surface and index finger on the volar surface. Additional stabilization can be achieved by holding client's hand against clinician's trunk.

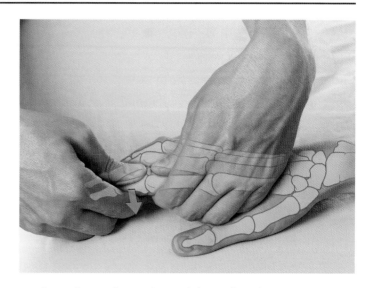

Mobilization: Clinician's mobilizing hand grips the proximal end of the more distal phalanx of the joint to be mobilized with thumb on the dorsal surface and index finger on the volar surface. The stabilizing hand holds the proximal phalanx in position while the mobilizing hand moves the distal phalanx in an anterior direction to elicit a ventral glide.

Goal of technique: To facilitate joint play in interphalangeal joints and aid in interphalangeal joint flexion.

Note: This is also a good technique for nourishment of the joint's articular cartilage.

TMC Distraction

Client position: Sitting with ulnar aspect of forearm on the treatment table. Keep trapeziometacarpal joint in resting open packed position.

Clinician position: Standing or sitting facing the trapeziometacarpal joint to be treated.

Stabilization: Clinician's proximal hand stabilizes by gripping the trapezium with thumb on the dorsal surface and index finger on the volar surface. Additional stabilization can be achieved by holding client's hand against clinician's trunk.

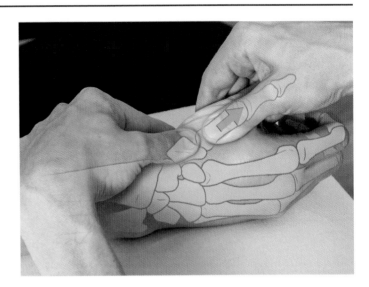

Mobilization: The clinician's mobilizing hand grabs the proximal metacarpal with thumb on the dorsal surface and index finger on the volar surface. Stabilizing hand holds the trapezium in position, while the mobilizing hand moves the metacarpal distally to create a distraction of the TMC joint.

Goals of technique: To promote joint play in the trapeziometacarpal joint and increase overall ROM.

Note: This technique is also good for articular nourishment to the thumb.

TMC Dorsal Glide

Client position: Sitting with ulnar aspect of forearm and hand on treatment table. Keep trapeziometacarpal joint in resting open packed position.

Clinician position: Standing or sitting facing the trapeziometacarpal joint to be treated.

Stabilization: Clinician's proximal hand stabilizes by gripping the trapezium with thumb on the palmar surface and index finger on the dorsal surface. Additional stabilization can be achieved by holding client's hand against clinician's trunk.

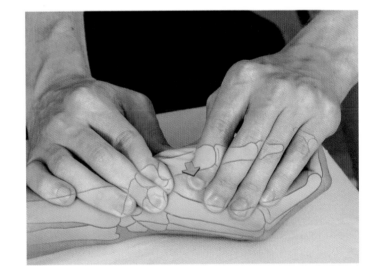

Mobilization: Clinician's mobilizing hand grabs the proximal metacarpal with thumb on the palmar surface and index finger on the dorsal surface. Stabilizing hand holds the trapezium in position, while the mobilizing hand moves the metacarpal in a dorsal direction to elicit a dorsal glide.

Goal of technique: To promote trapeziometacarpal joint abduction.

Note: This technique is also good for articular nourishment to the thumb.

TMC Ventral Glide

Client position: Sitting with ulnar aspect of forearm and hand on treatment table. Keep trapeziometacarpal joint in resting open packed position.

Clinician position: Standing or sitting facing the trapeziometacarpal joint to be treated.

Stabilization: Clinician's proximal hand stabilizes by gripping the trapezium with thumb on the palmar surface and index finger on the dorsal surface. Additional stabilization can be achieved by holding client's hand against clinician's trunk.

Mobilization: Clinician's mobilizing hand grabs the proximal metacarpal with thumb

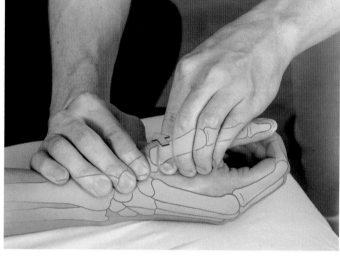

on the palmar surface and index finger on the dorsal surface. Stabilizing hand holds the trapezium in position, while the mobilizing hand moves the metacarpal in a volar direction to elicit a ventral glide.

Goal of technique: To promote trapeziometacarpal joint adduction.

Note: This technique is also good for articular nourishment to the thumb.

TMC Radial Glide

Client position: Sitting with ulnar aspect of forearm and hand on treatment table. Keep trapeziometacarpal joint in resting open packed position.

Clinician position: Standing or sitting facing the trapeziometacarpal joint to be treated.

Stabilization: Clinician's proximal hand stabilizes by gripping the trapezium with thumb on the palmar surface and index finger on the dorsal surface. Additional stabilization can be achieved by holding client's hand against clinician's trunk.

Mobilization: Clinician's mobilizing hand grabs the proximal metacarpal with thumb

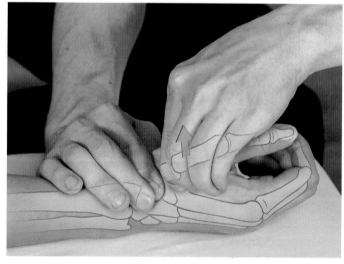

on the palmar surface and index finger on the dorsal surface. Stabilizing hand holds the trapezium in position, while the mobilizing hand moves the metacarpal toward the radius to impart a radial glide.

Goal of technique: To promote trapeziometacarpal joint extension.

Note: This technique is also good for articular nourishment to the thumb.

TMC Ulnar Glide

Client position: Sitting with ulnar aspect of forearm on treatment table. Keep trapeziometacarpal joint in resting open packed position.

Clinician position: Standing or sitting facing the trapeziometacarpal joint to be treated.

Stabilization: Clinician's proximal hand stabilizes by gripping the trapezium with thumb on the palmar surface and index finger on the dorsal surface. Additional stabilization can be achieved by holding client's hand against clinician's trunk.

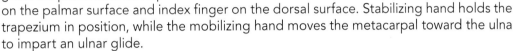

Mobilization: Clinician's mobilizing hand grabs the proximal metacarpal with thumb on the palmar surface and index finger on the dorsal surface. Stabilizing hand holds the trapezium in position, while the mobilizing hand moves the metacarpal toward the ulna to impart an ulnar glide.

Goal of technique: To promote trapeziometacarpal joint flexion.

Note: This technique is also good for articular nourishment to the thumb.

> Go to the web study guide and complete the case study for this chapter. The case study discusses a 55-year-old male with left wrist pain following a fall.

EVIDENCE FOR MANUAL THERAPY OF VARIOUS WRIST AND HAND PATHOLOGIES

Study	Clients	Intervention and comparison (if any)	Outcome(s)
Utilization of thrust and nonthrust mobilization for carpal tunnel syndrome: Grade C			
Tal-Akabi & Rushton, 2000 (Level 3b)	21 clients with symptoms of CTS	Clients were divided into 3 equal groups: (1) Control, (2) Median nerve mobilization, (3) Carpal mobilization	PRS was significantly different between treatment groups and the control group. No difference in PRS between treatment groups.
Utilization of thrust and nonthrust mobilization for Colles' fracture: Grade D			
Coyle & Robertson, 1998 (Level 4)	8 female clients postimmobilization Colles' fractures	Clients were randomly assigned to predesigned sets of treatment conditions. Two techniques: passive sustained stretch and oscillations for 6 treatments.	Oscillating joint mobilization was more effective in decreasing pain compared to passive stretching. Both were effective for improving AROM.
Utilization of thrust and nonthrust mobilization for MCP joint: Grade C			
Randall et al., 1992 (Level 3b)	18 clients postimmobilization following a metacarpal fracture	Clients were randomly assigned to a joint mobilization group or control group. Joint mobilization included distraction and volar glides. Treatment was provided 3 times for 1 week.	AROM and joint stiffness was significantly improved in the treatment group as compared to the control group.
Utilization of thrust and nonthrust mobilization for CMC OA: Grade A			
Villafañe et al., 2013 (Level 1b)	60 clients with CMC OA; 90% were females	Clients were randomly assigned to receive a multimodal manual treatment approach that included joint mobilization, neural mobilization, and exercise, or a sham intervention, for 12 sessions over 4 weeks. Joint mobilization was distraction with posterior-anterior glides.	A combination of joint mobilization, neural mobilization, and exercise was more beneficial in treating pain than a sham intervention in clients with CMC joint OA.

CTS = carpal tunnel syndrome; PRS = pain rating scale; AROM = active range of motion; MCP = metacarpophalangeal joint; CMC = carpometacarpal joint; OA = osteoarthritis

PART IV

Mobilization and Manipulation of the Lower Extremity

Part IV consists of 4 chapters that cover thrust and nonthrust techniques for the lower extremity: hip, knee, ankle, and foot. Chapter 10 covers the hip joint, a multiplanar articulation between the femur and acetabulum. Techniques are described for distraction and all planes of hip movement: flexion, extension, abduction, adduction, and internal and external rotation. The knee joint complex is presented in chapter 11. Knee techniques are divided by joint articulation and include the tibiofemoral joint, patellofemoral joint, and superior tibiofibular joint. Techniques are described for improving the primary motion of knee flexion and extension. Chapter 12 covers the ankle joint complex consisting of the distal tibiofibular joint and talocrural joint. The final chapter of this section is chapter 13 on the foot. Because of the multiple joints that make up the foot, numerous techniques are presented.

Explicit instructions for all techniques are included with detailed overlaid photos to help the clinician with technique precision. The techniques described include multiple positions and potential modifications to accommodate clients who may have difficulty achieving a particular position. Current evidence for techniques is included in a table at the end of each chapter.

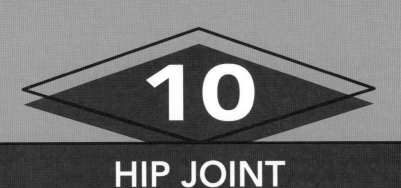

HIP JOINT

The hip joint is a weight-bearing, synovial ball-and-socket joint that can sustain very large forces through its joint surfaces. Similar to the shoulder, open kinetic chain motion encompasses a convex femoral head moving on a relatively fixed concave acetabulum. In weight bearing, however, these roles reverse, with the convex femoral head as the relatively fixed surface and the acetabulum now the moving surface. This type of motion is common in many daily activities and sports, such as pivoting or twisting motions (e.g., golf swing, batting, turning a corner when walking, bending over to tie your shoes when sitting). Understanding the anatomy and kinematics of the hip joint, both weight bearing and non–weight bearing, is crucial to properly treating the client with hip joint–related dysfunction when mobilization is a key part of their treatment.

Anatomy

The hip, or femoroacetabular joint, is a ball-and-socket synovial joint, similar to the shoulder joint. Other similarities between the shoulder and hip joint exist in anatomy and joint kinematics. Unlike the shoulder, the hip is primarily weight bearing and is less complex with respect to the number of bones and joint articulations. The hip joint is inherently a stable joint, yet has a moderate amount of mobility. The hip joint also is designed to encounter large forces transmitted through it. The bones encompassing the hip joint are the pelvis (ilium, ischium, pubis) and proximal femur. Despite its relative simplicity, the hip joint functions as the primary stabilizing structure for the lower extremity.

The hip joint consists of 1 single articulation between the femoral head and the acetabulum, referred to as the femoroacetabular joint (figure 10.1). This joint is a diarthrodial spheroidal joint, more commonly known as a synovial ball-and-socket joint. The joint articulation occurs between the aspherical (convex) head of the femur and the concave acetabulum. This articulation is primarily on the crescent-shaped lunate surface of the acetabulum. This articular surface is covered with articular cartilage and lubricated with synovial fluid to reduce friction. The nonarticulating surface is called the acetabular fossa. Static stabilization occurs via the depth of the acetabulum, the spiraling nature of the joint capsule, fibrous acetabular labrum, and femoroacetabular ligaments. Unlike the limited congruency in the shoulder, the acetabulum typically encompasses more than half of the head of the femur, providing significant stability. The dynamic stability of the femoroacetabular joint is provided primarily by the gluteal and other muscles acting on the joint.

The soft tissue structures around the hip, especially hip joint–related muscles, are some of the largest in the body. Three primary extra-articular ligaments are thickenings of the hip joint capsule (figure 10.2). While various hip motions make these different ligaments taut, they are all taut with hip extension.

The gluteal muscles are some of the largest and most important musculature of the hip joint (figure 10.3). The gluteus maximus has principal functions of hip extension, abduction, and external rotation (as well as decelerating hip flexion, adduction, and internal rotation in a closed kinetic chain position), whereas the gluteus medius' principal function in the open kinetic chain is hip abduction and, in a closed kinetic chain position, deceleration of contralateral pelvic drop. The primary anterior hip joint muscle are the iliacus and psoas (or commonly referred to as iliopsoas) muscles (figure 10.4). Functioning together, these muscles primarily flex the hip.

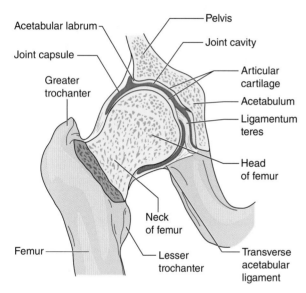

Figure 10.1 Femoroacetabular joint.

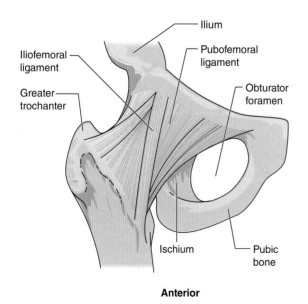

Anterior

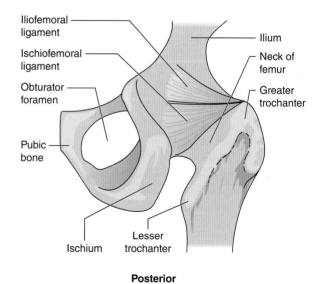

Posterior

Figure 10.2 Primary ligaments about the hip.

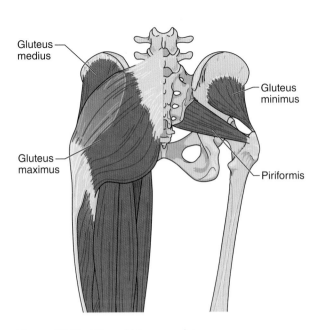

Figure 10.3 Gluteal hip musculature.

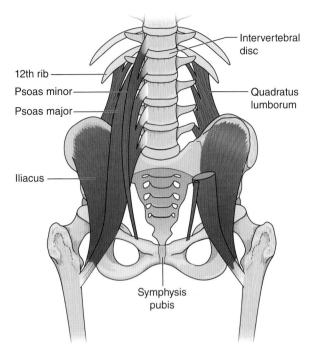

Figure 10.4 Iliopsoas hip musculature.

Joint Kinematics

Motion at the femoroacetabular joint occurs in all 3 planes, occurring between the convex femoral head and the concave acetabulum. The axis of motion in all 3 planes is in the center of the femoral head, indicating almost pure spin in these motions. Arthrokinematically, the motion of the hip is primarily a spin of the femoral head within the acetabulum, accompanied by slight gliding (figure 10.5). The femoroacetabular joint anatomy and congruency limit significant translation between the joint surfaces.

Open Kinetic Chain Kinematics

Hip flexion and extension occur in the sagittal plane through a medial/lateral axis. Similar to the shoulder, both flexion and extension are primarily a spinning of the joint (femoral head) along the articulating surface (in this case, the acetabulum). The physiological motion of hip flexion, though, is accompanied by a small amount of posterior and inferior accessory motion of the femoral head on the acetabulum. Conversely, the physiological motion of hip extension is accompanied by a small amount of anterior and superior accessory motion of the femoral head on the acetabulum. Again, however, the accessory motion required for both

of these physiological motions is the femoral head spinning on the acetabulum.

Rotation movements in the hip joint occur in the transverse plane through a superoinferior axis. External rotation in the hip joint is accomplished by anterior glide of the femoral head. As the femur externally rotates, the convex humeral head rolls posteriorly and glides anteriorly. With the hip flexed to 90°, the femoral head glides superiorly with external rotation. In a non-weight-bearing position, internal rotation is accomplished by posterior glide of the femoral head. The convex femoral head performs anterior rolling and posterior gliding on the concave acetabulum.

Hip abduction and adduction occur in the frontal plane around an anteroposterior axis. The center of rotation during abduction and adduction occurs through the center of the femoral head. As the convex femoral head rolls superiorly during abduction, a concomitant inferior glide motion occurs. Because of the geometry of the femoral head, if the hip is flexed close to 90°, the arthrokinematics change. If the hip is flexed to 90°, the femoral head will glide anteriorly with abduction. During hip adduction, the femoral head rolls inferiorly, as there is a superior gliding motion. With the hip flexed to 90°, the femoral head glides posteriorly to achieve adduction.

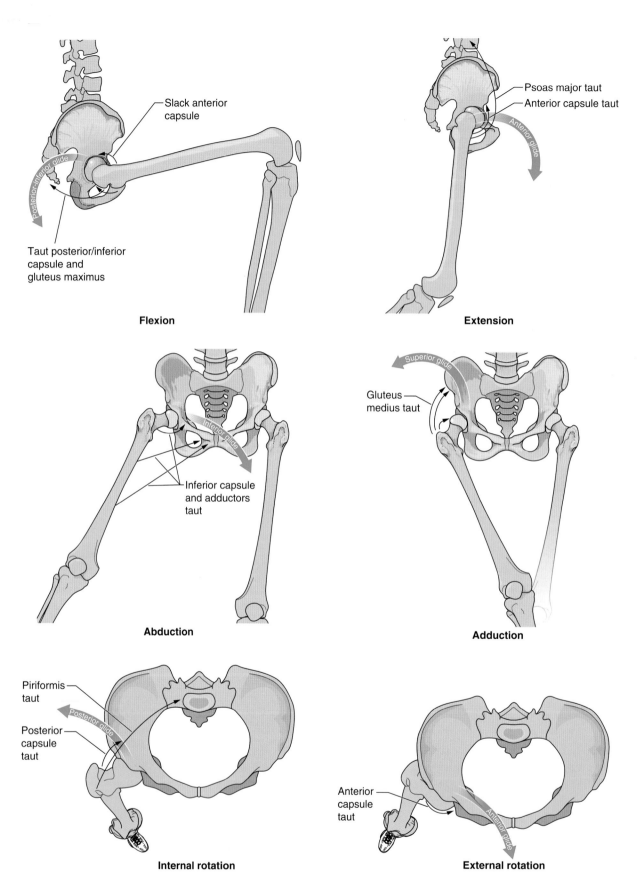

Flexion

Slack anterior capsule

Taut posterior/inferior capsule and gluteus maximus

Posterior-inferior glide

Extension

Psoas major taut
Anterior capsule taut

Anterior glide

Abduction

Inferior glide

Inferior capsule and adductors taut

Adduction

Superior glide

Gluteus medius taut

Internal rotation

Piriformis taut

Posterior capsule taut

Posterior glide

External rotation

Anterior capsule taut

Anterior glide

Figure 10.5 Open kinetic chain kinematic (femur on acetabulum of pelvis) of the hip joint. Sagittal plane: flexion and extension. Frontal plane: abduction and adduction. Horizontal plane: internal rotation and external rotation.

Closed Kinetic Chain Kinematics

Closed kinetic chain kinematics describes the pelvis (via the acetabulum) moving on a relatively fixed femur. This motion requires the femur to be relatively fixed, thus in a weight-bearing position. The motions can still occur in all 3 planes of motion as they do with open kinetic chain motion.

◆ *Flexion.* In standing, to bend forward as if to touch your toes, the pelvis rotates anteriorly on the fixed femur (concave moving on convex). Lumbar spine movement will also correlate with this motion with the lumbar spine moving into flexion.

◆ *Extension.* With the foot on the ground, relative hip extension requires the pelvis to rotate posteriorly on the fixed femur. Lumbar spine movement will also correlate with this motion with the lumbar spine moving into extension.

◆ *Internal rotation.* In stance, internal rotation is achieved by the acetabulum spinning about the femoral head toward the side of rotation (figure 10.6). For right lower-extremity internal rotation, the pelvis will rotate to the right. An example: for a right-handed golfer starting in a neutral position and moving to the backswing, the right hip would be in internal rotation at the end of the backswing.

◆ *External rotation.* With the foot fixed, external rotation is achieved by the acetabulum spinning about the femoral head opposite the side of rotation (figure 10.6). For left lower-extremity external rotation, the pelvis will rotate to the right. An example: for a right-handed golfer starting in a neutral position and moving to the backswing, the left hip would be in external rotation at the end of the backswing.

◆ *Abduction.* In a weight-bearing state, the concave acetabulum glides toward the opposite pelvis, with the contralateral side of the pelvis hiking.

◆ *Adduction.* In a weight-bearing state, the concave acetabulum glides inferiorly toward the ipsilateral femur, with the contralateral side of the pelvis dropping (figure 10.7).

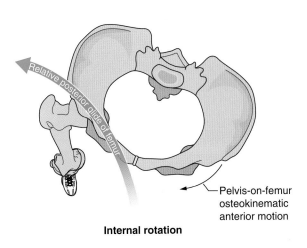

Internal rotation

Pelvis-on-femur osteokinematic anterior motion

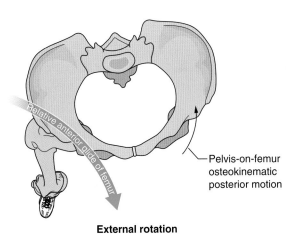

External rotation

Pelvis-on-femur osteokinematic posterior motion

Figure 10.6 Pelvis on femur (closed kinetic chain) transverse plane motion.

Clinical Tip

When assessing or treating the hip joint, it is important for the clinician to understand the kinematics of the joint and whether the symptoms are provoked primarily in the weight-bearing or non-weight-bearing position. The techniques described in this chapter are primarily non–weight bearing, but the reader should view the self-mobilization section for ideas on techniques to implement in the weight-bearing position.

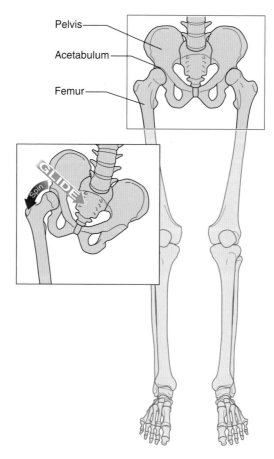

Figure 10.7 Pelvis on femur (closed kinetic chain) frontal plane adduction motion.

HIP JOINT ARTHROLOGY

Articular surfaces	Closed packed position	Resting position	Capsular pattern	ROM norms	End-feel
Femoroacetabular					
OKC Moving surface is femur (convex); stable surface is acetabulum (concave) **CKC** Moving surface is acetabulum (concave) moving on stationary femur (convex)	**Ligamentous** Full extension, abduction, internal rotation **Bony** 90° flexion, slight abduction, slight external rotation	30° flexion 30° abduction Slight external rotation	Flexion, abduction, internal rotation	Flexion: 140° with knee flexed Extension: 20° Internal rotation: 45° External rotation: 45° Abduction: 40° Adduction: 25°	Firm for all motions

OKC = open kinetic chain; CKC = closed kinetic chain

Indirect (Longitudinal) Distraction

VIDEO 10.1 **in the web study guide shows this technique.**

Client position: Supine with leg relaxed.

Clinician position: Standing facing client's hip to be treated.

Stabilization: Client's body on treatment table serves as stabilization.

Mobilization: Clinician places hip in resting position. *(a)* Distraction force in caudal direction imposed through both hands and leaning body back. Clinician grabs client's leg proximal to knee with both hands, placing client's leg between clinician's arm and trunk for improved purchase. *(b)* To increase leverage, and likely increase amount of distraction force, a more distal purchase just above the medial and lateral malleoli can be used. *(c)* Additionally, use of a belt in a figure 8 format can improve clinician's ability to purchase.

Goals of technique: To help with multiplanar joint mobility limitations and pain with weight bearing.

Notes: This technique can also be used as a thrust technique. The clinician grasps above the client's bilateral malleoli. The client is stabilized either with *(d)* a mobilization belt strapped to the treatment table or bedsheet proximally in groin and held by another clinician. Positioning is the same as described in the preceding section. The clinician takes up the slack in the joint and performs a high-velocity, low-amplitude thrust.

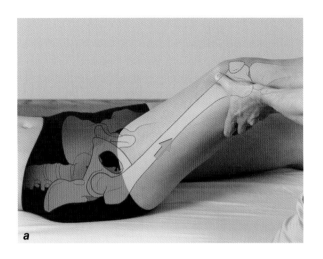

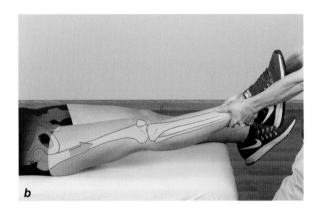

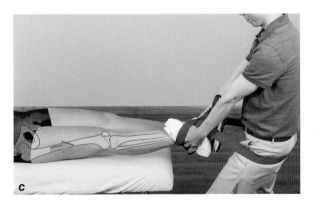

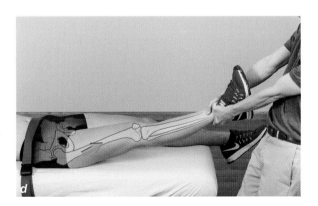

Indirect (Longitudinal) Distraction via Knee Purchase

Client position: Supine with hip to be treated in 50° of hip flexion with foot flat on treatment table.

Clinician position: Sitting on the foot of the extremity to be treated, facing client.

Stabilization: Client's body weight and clinician's body weight on client's foot provide stabilization. Client may grasp treatment table (at the side, not overhead) for additional stabilization. Additionally, skin contact on the table can provide stabilization.

Mobilization: Clinician hooks forearm (maximally pronated) closest to midline of client underneath client's knee and grasps opposite forearm. The other hand is placed on the anterior/medial surface of the distal femur. Both of clinician's arms should

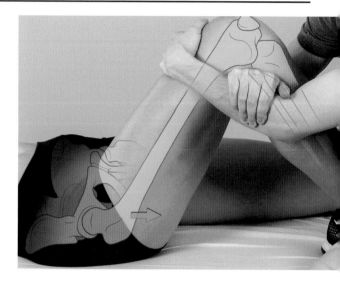

be maximally horizontally adducted (pull both elbows toward each other) to limit pull from arms. Clinician then applies a distraction force to the hip by leaning his or her body backward.

Goals of technique: To help with multiplanar joint mobility limitations and pain with weight bearing (load sensitivity). This mobilization is also effective for increasing general hip motion.

Notes: The degree of hip abduction and flexion can vary. Skin contact on the treatment table can prevent the whole client's body from sliding down the table. The client's other leg should be relaxed and straight.

Lateral Distraction

Client position: Supine with leg positioned on clinician's shoulder.

Clinician position: Standing next to leg to be treated, facing client's hip.

Stabilization: Client's body weight serves to stabilize. A belt around client's pelvis and table may be used for additional stabilization.

Mobilization: Clinician places both hands on the anterior/medial surface of the proximal thigh and, with body weight, mobilizes the femoral head in an inferior/lateral direction (perpendicular to the acetabular surface).

Goals of technique: To help with multiplanar joint mobility limitations and pain with weight bearing (load sensitivity); to increase general hip motion and stretching all fibers of the hip capsule in a lateral direction.

Notes: The mobilization might be most effective if the clinician's hands are placed as close to the hip joint as possible. The clinician's shoulder should be as close to the client's thigh and posterior knee as possible. This technique can also be supplemented with the use of a belt around client's proximal thigh and around the buttocks.

Inferior Glide

VIDEO 10.2 **in the web study guide shows this technique.**

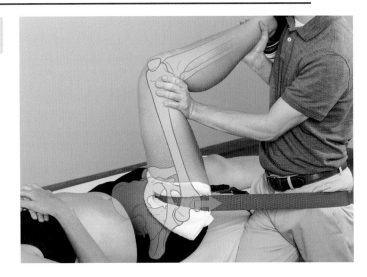

Client position: Supine with hip to be treated flexed to 90°.

Clinician position: Standing inferior to the hip to be treated. A mobilization belt is wrapped around client's proximal thigh and clinician.

Stabilization: Client's body weight in addition to clinician's hands on the posterior distal thigh serve to stabilize.

Mobilization: Clinician mobilizes hip in an inferior direction through the belt, using a shift of body weight.

Goals of technique: To treat accessory motion limitations in flexion; to decrease pinching pain in anterior hip; to stretch primarily the inferior capsule.

Notes: If the client can tolerate full knee flexion with a little overpressure, the clinician can grasp bilateral hands over the belt, place shoulder (deltopectoral groove) on client's anterior knee, and use a scooping motion when performing this technique. The clinician pushes his or her buttocks toward the client's feet and the ceiling (along with the belt) and shoulders forward and toward the client to impart an inferior/anterior glide of proximal femoral head with hip flexion.

Anterior Glide in Prone

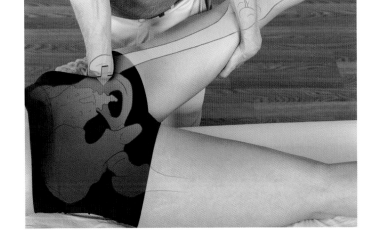

Client position: Prone with leg to be treated beyond edge of treatment table.

Clinician position: Standing at side of client near hip to be treated, facing client.

Stabilization: The stabilizing hand holds client's thigh proximal to knee. Client's body weight also serves to stabilize.

Mobilization: The mobilizing hand is positioned on the posterior surface of the proximal thigh and mobilizes the femur in an anterior direction using broad hand contact.

Goals of technique: To treat accessory motion restrictions in extension, external rotation, and abduction at near hip neutral or in extension. This technique will likely impart force on the anterior capsule and psoas muscle.

Notes: As with all relevant hip mobilization techniques, position the mobilizing hand on the femur as close to the hip joint as possible. This mobilization can be applied in positions approaching the joint's end range of extension for a more aggressive technique.

Clinical tip: The clinician should be cognizant of the ligamentous closed packed position of the hip joint (full extension, abduction, internal rotation).

Anterior Glide in Modified Prone

Client position: Prone with upper body supported on treatment table at the level of the anterior superior iliac crest. The leg to be treated is supported between clinician's thighs just above the knees. The contralateral limb rests on ground for support.

Clinician position: Standing posterior to client with leg to be treated between distal thighs.

Stabilization: Leg between clinician's thighs and client's contact with treatment table provides stabilization.

Mobilization: Clinician places web spaces of both hands (or palms of both hands) against the proximal posterior thigh (as close to hip joint as possible) and mobilizes in an anterior direction using body weight through extended elbows.

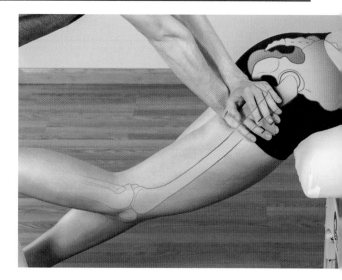

Goals of technique: To treat accessory motion restrictions in extension, external rotation, and abduction at short of neutral hip flexion. The force will likely be imparted on the anterior capsule and psoas muscle.

Note: This mobilization is a less aggressive treatment because the hip is flexed nearer to its resting position.

Anterior Glide in Prone FABER Position

 VIDEO 10.3 **in the web study guide shows this technique.**

Client position: Prone with hip to be treated in a position of flexion, abduction, and external rotation (FABER), with knee off edge of treatment table and flexed. The client's pelvis should be parallel to the table.

Clinician position: Standing to side of client, bracing client's knee with thigh.

Stabilization: Client's body weight serves to stabilize. A belt around client's pelvis and table may be used for additional stabilization.

Mobilization: Clinician places web spaces of both hands against the proximal posterior thigh

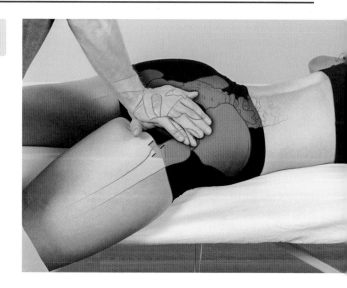

or hands as shown and mobilizes in an anterior or anterior/medial direction using body weight through extended elbows.

Goals of technique: To treat accessory motion restrictions in extension, external rotation, and abduction, especially relative to the FABER test position of the hip joint.

Notes: The client with very limited mobility in the supine FABER position should be moved as close to the edge of the treatment table as possible to ensure the pelvis is parallel to the table and to decrease the stress on the femur being mobilized.

Posterior Glide in Resting Position

Client position: Supine with side to be treated near edge of treatment table.

Clinician position: Standing to side of client, supporting client's leg between trunk and stabilizing hand.

Stabilization: Client's body against treatment table serves to stabilize.

Mobilization: Clinician positions the mobilizing hand on the anterior surface of the proximal thigh with forearm pronated and mobilizes the femur in a posterior-lateral direction. Clinician should keep the mobilizing arm elbow completely straight to impart force of body weight through the arm.

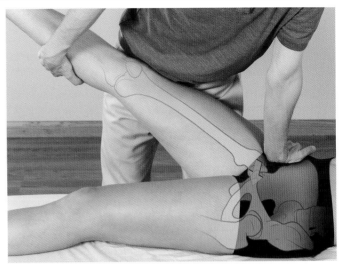

Goals of technique: Treat accessory motion restrictions in flexion, internal rotation, and adduction at 30° of hip flexion (or near resting position). This technique is also effective as a pain modulation technique for clients who have a pain-dominant (versus stiffness-dominant) presentation.

Notes: Varying degrees of hip flexion may be used. It is important to be able to monitor the client's reaction to this (and any) technique by not turning your back to the client when performing the technique.

Posterior Glide in Hook-Lying

VIDEO 10.4 **in the web study guide shows this technique.**

Client position: Supine with hip to be treated in approximately 50° of hip flexion; foot flat on treatment table.

Clinician position: Standing on opposite side to be treated. Clinician places hip to be treated in a comfortable position of flexion, adduction, and internal rotation.

Stabilization: Client's body against treatment table serves as stabilization.

Mobilization: Clinician places both hands on top of the knee to be treated and mobilizes through the long axis of the femur in a posterior-lateral direction.

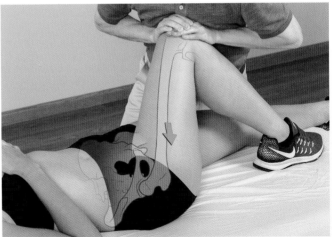

Goals of technique: To treat accessory motion restrictions in flexion, internal rotation, and adduction at 90° hip flexion. This technique is also effective for clients with complaints in positions similar to hip impingement and squatting.

Notes: The mobilization can be made more aggressive by grabbing the client's posterior pelvis, grabbing the side of the treatment table, or adding more flexion, adduction, and/or internal rotation to the hip.

Clinical tip: The greater the force requirement, the more likely you would grab either the client's pelvis or treatment table.

Direct Lateral Glide

Client position: Supine with hip to be treated in 60° of hip flexion with foot flat on treatment table.

Clinician position: Standing next to the leg to be treated facing client.

Stabilization: Client's body weight serves as stabilization. Clinician also uses his or her deltopectoral groove against the lateral aspect of client's knee as a counterforce.

Mobilization: Clinician places both hands on the medial surface of the proximal thigh and (using body weight) mobilizes the femur away from the acetabulum in a lateral direction.

Goals of technique: To help with adduction and multiplanar joint mobility limitations; to alleviate pain with weight bearing (load sensitivity); and to impart direct lateral stretch of entire hip joint capsule.

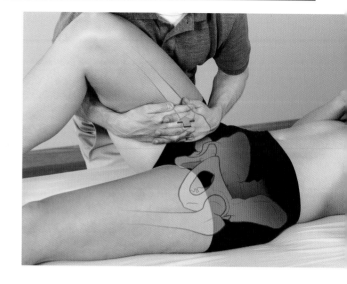

Notes: The mobilization might be most effective if the clinician's hands are placed as close to the hip joint as possible. A belt around client's proximal thigh and clinician's buttocks (similar to lateral glide internal rotation mobilization technique) is also suggested.

Lateral Glide Internal Rotation Motion

Client position: Supine with hip to be treated flexed to 90°.

Clinician position: Standing lateral to hip to be treated. A mobilization belt is wrapped around client's proximal thigh and clinician. Client's leg is held at ankle in any desired degree of internal rotation with 1 hand while the other provides a medial counterforce against the lateral knee.

Stabilization: Client's body weight in addition to clinician's hand on the lateral knee serve as stabilization.

Mobilization: Clinician mobilizes the hip in a lateral direction through the belt using a shift of body weight as the hip is internally rotated either passively or actively (depending on goal of treatment).

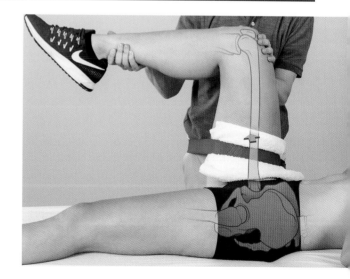

Goals of technique: This mobilization treats limitations in hip internal rotation and adduction, as well as general hip limitations. It also likely imparts a lateral stretch of the entire hip joint capsule.

Notes: The clinician's shoulders should always stay parallel to the client's shin. Monitor for trunk compensatory motion and control as tolerated.

Indirect Technique: Posterior-Lateral Glide

Client position: Prone with knee of the extremity to be treated flexed to 90°.

Clinician position: Standing next to hip to be treated with 1 hand holding the extremity's ankle to control desired degree of internal rotation.

Stabilization: Client's body against treatment table serves as stabilization.

Mobilization: The mobilizing hand is placed over the dorsal aspect of the ilium just lateral to the sacrum and provides an anterior/medial mobilization to the pelvis, essentially performing a posterior-lateral mobilization to the femur.

Goals of technique: This mobilization treats internal rotation limitations of the hip indirectly. An indirect technique such as this one (while not likely commonly necessary) might be required when client cannot tolerate pressure or force directly at the hip joint.

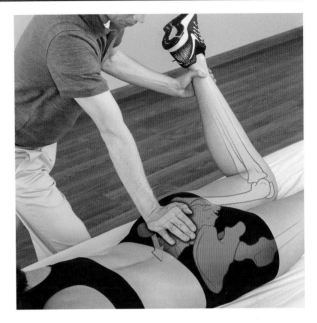

Notes: The clinician should maintain full elbow extension and use his or her body weight to perform the technique. This is not a good technique for clients with co-existing sacroiliac joint pathology.

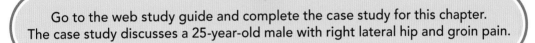

Go to the web study guide and complete the case study for this chapter. The case study discusses a 25-year-old male with right lateral hip and groin pain.

EVIDENCE FOR MANUAL THERAPY OF VARIOUS HIP JOINT PATHOLOGIES

Study	Clients	Intervention and comparison (if any)	Outcome(s)
Utilization of thrust and nonthrust mobilization for osteoarthritis: Grade B			
Beumer et al., 2016 (Level 1a)	3 studies	Various MT +/– exercise vs. control Various MT +/– exercise vs. control MT + exercise vs. exercise	MT +/– exercise was favored over control. MT +/– exercise slightly favored over control. MT favored over exercise. Overall recommendation from study: limited to no support for MT for hip OA for short-term benefit, although study heterogeneity was significant.
Sampath et al., 2015 (Level 1a)	7 studies (886 clients)	Various grouping of MT and exercise combined vs. control groups	Low-quality evidence supporting MT and exercise for pain, quality of life, and improvement in physical function posttreatment and follow-up.
Romeo et al., 2013 (Level 1a)	10 studies	Various grouping of MT and exercise combined vs. control groups	Moderate evidence suggests improvement in function for use of MT and exercise, while limited evidence supports MT and exercise for pain and quality of life.
Bennell et al., 2014 (Level 1b)	102 community subjects (49 in treatment group, 53 in sham control)	Education, advice, manual therapy, home exercise, and gait aid as needed—10 visits to PT Sham = inactive ultrasound and inert gel-10 visits to PT	No difference between groups at 13 weeks for self-reported pain (VAS) or function (WOMAC). Single-leg balance greater in intervention group.
Pinto et al., 2011 (Level 1b)	206 clients with diagnosed OA	MT, exercise therapy, and control group	MT and exercise groups were more cost effective than usual care control group.
Hoeksma et al., 2004 (Level 1b)	109 clients diagnosed with hip OA (56 for MT and 53 for exercise)	MT (stretching of hip, traction of hip joint, and traction thrust technique) Exercise focus on improving ROM and strength, along with walking endurance	After 5 weeks, success rate of MT was 81% versus 50% for exercise. MT not more effective than exercise in those clients with highly limited function, ROM, or high pain levels. Improvements in function declined after 5 weeks of stopping interventions. Some improvement lasted up to 29 weeks for clients in the MT group.
Utilization of thrust and nonthrust mobilization for femoroacetabular impingement: Grade C			
Wright et al., 2016 (Level 2b)	15 clients with diagnosed FAI	MT and exercise with advice and home program vs. advice and home program	Both groups significantly improved in pain. Group differences for changes in pain or physical function were not significant.
Reiman and Matheson, 2013 (Level 5)	NA	NA	Clinical review and technique suggestion article based on clinical findings of hip joint limitations in clients diagnosed with FAI (Diamond et al., 2015).
Utilization of thrust and nonthrust mobilization for hip instability: Grade F			
Enseki et al., 2014 (Level 5)	NA	NA	CPG recommending "Joint mobilization, except for pain modulation, is contraindicated in individuals classified as hypermobile."

PT = physical therapy; MT = manual therapy; OA = osteoarthritis; VAS = visual analog scale; WOMAC = Western Ontario and McMaster Universities Arthritis Index; NA = not applicable; CPG = clinical practice guideline; FAI = femoroacetabular impingement

11

KNEE JOINT

LEARNING OBJECTIVES

After completing this chapter, you will be able to do the following:

◆ Describe the bony and soft tissue anatomy of the knee complex

◆ Describe the joint kinematics of the knee joint

◆ Describe positioning, movements, and reasoning behind knee mobilization

◆ Identify evidence supporting joint mobilization techniques for the knee

Although it appears to be a fairly simple joint, the knee is much more complex than previously thought. It is a complex of 2 different joints: the tibiofemoral joint and the patellofemoral joint. Because the knee is the confluence of the 2 longest bones in the body it has incredible stresses applied to it that are not seen anywhere else in the human body. Unlike its upper extremity counterpart, the elbow, the knee must function in a closed chain fashion a large amount of the time. Therefore, weight-bearing forces are born and transferred from distal to proximal through the foot to the knee and eventually to the hip and lower back. The amount of forces placed on the knee during running, cutting, and jumping are tremendous. The knee must accomplish a delicate balance of stability and mobility to function during activities of daily living, as well as vocational and recreational activities.

Injuries can occur at both the tibiofemoral joint and the patellofemoral joint. Tibiofemoral injuries include ligament and articular cartilage and meniscus lesions. These can cause knee pain, swelling, and feelings of or actual joint instability. Injuries to the patellofemoral joint include overuse injuries as well as traumatic injuries, including quadriceps and patellar rupture and patellar fractures. Any of these forms of injury can lead to disability and loss of normal daily function, a tragic circumstance given that normal gait and mobility depend on a functional knee.

Anatomy

The knee joint is comprised of 2 far different joints: the larger tibiofemoral joint and the smaller patellofemoral joint. The tibiofemoral joint is the largest joint of the body and allows a large degree of flexion and extension mobility and less rotation motion. The patellofemoral joint is comprised of the patella, the largest sesamoid bone in the body, and the trochlea of the distal femur. Each of these 2 joints has unique features, and a full understanding of the anatomy and kinematics of each joint is needed to properly treat clients with limitations of knee mobility.

Tibiofemoral Joint

The tibiofemoral joint consists of the proximal tibia and the distal trochlea surface of the femur (figure 11.1). Between these 2 bones is an interposed meniscus. Overall tibiofemoral alignment is determined by the position of the hip. In healthy subjects, the hip runs medial and distal from its proximal end to the distal knee. This angle of inclination is approximately 125°. Although the axis of this motion runs through the center of the femur, the result does not alter the position of the femoral condyles because the medial condyle extends further than the lateral. In this manner, the condyles are able to rest horizontally on the proximal tibia. Most humans exhibit a slight valgus angulation of 5° to 10°, termed genu valgum (or "knock-kneed"). This angle becomes pathologic if it exceeds 10°. When the tibiofemoral angle is angled medially in

the frontal plane, it is known as genu varum (or "bow-legged"). This angle becomes excessive or pathological if greater than 5°. Potentially harmful compressive forces can be placed on the lateral compartment in those with genu valgum, and on the medial side in those with genu varum.

Patellofemoral Joint

The patellofemoral joint is an incongruent joint on the anterior surface of the knee that is formed between the anterior femur and the posterior patellar surface. Because the trochlear surface of the femur is fairly shallow, the patella does not fit deeply into the patellar sulcus. The lateral trochlea extends further anterior than that of the medial, suggesting it might be helpful for restraining lateral translational forces of the patella (figure 11.2). The patella is primarily dependent on dynamic stability provided by the quadriceps muscles and iliotibial band, while static stability is afforded through patellar retinacular tissues, the knee capsule, and medial and lateral patellofemoral ligaments.

Muscles

Muscles surrounding the knee are crucial to assist with dynamic control of the limb. These muscles are divided into quadriceps and hamstring groupings.

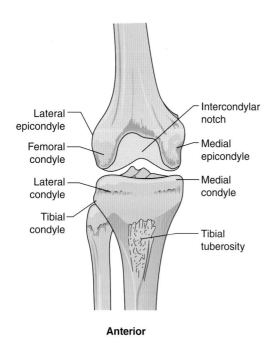

Anterior

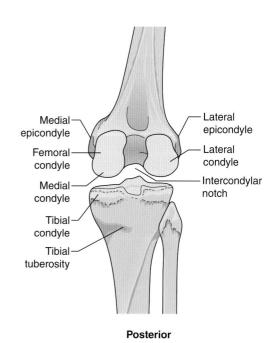

Posterior

Figure 11.1 Tibiofemoral joint and respective bony anatomy.

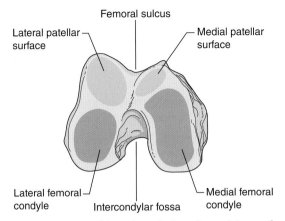

Femoral sulcus

Lateral patellar surface

Medial patellar surface

Lateral femoral condyle

Intercondylar fossa

Medial femoral condyle

Figure 11.2 Trochlear (patellar) and condylar surface of the distal femur. This figure clearly shows that the lateral patellar surface extends further anterior than that of the medial.

Quadriceps Group

The knee extensors consist of a group of muscles known as the quadriceps. This group consists of the rectus femoris, vastus lateralis, vastus medialis, and vastus intermedius. The rectus femoris arises from the anterior inferior iliac spine, whereas the other 3 vasti muscles arise from the femur. The rectus runs distally to blend with the remaining vasti muscles, which collectively attach to the quadriceps tendon that attaches to the proximal patella. A portion of this tendon continues distally to become the patellar tendon and eventually the patellar ligament to attach distally at the tibial tuberosity. The vastus lateralis is the lateral most vasti. It is a large and thick muscle that arises from the intertrochanteric line, the greater trochanter, the gluteal tuberosity, the lateral linea aspera, and the lateral intermuscular septum. As with the remaining vasti muscles, it too runs distally to blend into the lateral portion of the patellar tendon. The vastus medialis covers the medial portion of the knee and arises from the medial intermuscular septum, the intertrochanteric line, and the spiral line. This muscle also blends with the rectus and vastus lateralis to attach at the quadriceps tendon. Finally, the vastus intermedius is a deep vasti that lies under the rectus femoris. It arises from the lateral surface of the upper two-thirds of the shaft of the femur, the distal portion of the lateral intermuscular septum, and the lateral lip of the linea aspera. It joins deep to the other vasti to attach to the quadriceps tendon.

The vasti muscles all arise from the femur, so they extend only the knee; however, the rectus

femoris crosses both the hip and the knee and is therefore biarticular, with actions of knee extension and hip flexion.

Hamstring Group

The primary motion at the tibiofemoral joint is flexion and extension in the sagittal plane, so the musculature is easily divided into knee flexors or knee extensors. The knee flexors are the hamstrings, gracillis, and sartorius, whereas the knee extensors consist of the quadriceps muscle group.

The largest hamstring knee flexor is the biceps femoris, found on the posterior-lateral portion of the thigh. This muscle has 2 heads, 1 short and 1 long. The short head arises from the lateral lip of the linea aspera and the lateral intermuscular septum, whereas the long head arises from the ischial tuberosity. As the 2 heads progress inferiorly they join together at about the level of the posterior midthigh. They both then proceed to attach at the fibular head, the fascia of the lower leg, the lateral collateral ligament, and the lateral capsule of the knee.

The medial hamstrings include the semimembranosus and the semitendinosus, which arise at the ischial tuberosity. The semitendinosus, as its name implies, remains tendinous for a longer portion of its length as compared to the more muscular semimembranosus. Each of these muscles attaches distally to the fascia of the lower leg and the proximal portion of the medial tibia.

Because all of the flexor muscles are biarticular they can flex the knee and extend the hip. During open kinetic chain movements, the hamstrings collectively flex the knee and extend the hip. However, in closed kinetic chain activities the hamstrings provide a restraint of the pelvis and trunk to forward movements. When the medial or lateral hamstrings contract individually they can create a rotation moment at the tibia. Isolated contraction of the medial hamstrings with the knee flexed can create medial tibial rotation, whereas an isolated contraction of the lateral biceps femoris creates lateral tibial rotation.

Additional Anatomical Structures

Additional anatomical structures are discussed to be all inclusive regarding anatomy surrounding the knee. These additional structures include the joint capsule, fat pads, menisci, and ligaments.

Each of these structures has unique functions in knee anatomy.

Joint Capsule

A large joint capsule surrounds the entire knee joint, including both the tibiofemoral joint and the patellofemoral joint. This external capsule is fibrous on the outside and composed of synovial tissue on its inner surface. The posterior portion of the capsule ends much more abruptly than its anterior portion, which extends about a hand's breadth superiorly above the joint line. The superior portion of the capsule is placed on tension during knee flexion motion, and placed on slack during extension. The posterior capsule, therefore, is slack with knee flexion and taut during knee extension. Due to the extreme amount of motion that occurs at the knee, the capsule is reinforced by multiple muscles, tendons, and ligaments.

Infrapatellar Fat Pads

An extensive fat pad extends superiorly beneath the patellar tendon and separates it from the tibia, providing cushion to the patellar tendon, and is thought to help lubricate it. Known as Hoffa's pads, these tissues can be a source of anterior knee pain.

Menisci

Due to the incongruence of the tibiofemoral bony structures, an interposed meniscus increases joint congruity. The meniscus are fibrocartilaginous discs that enhance joint congruence, distribute weight-bearing forces, reduce friction, and serve as shock absorbers (figure 11.3). The menisci cover one-half to two-thirds of the superior surface of the tibia. The medial meniscus is C-shaped and has a large diameter since the medial tibial plateau is larger than that of the lateral. The medial meniscus has a firm attachment to the medial collateral ligament and medial capsule. The lateral meniscus is more circular shaped and has no attachment to the lateral collateral ligament. The lateral meniscus covers a larger surface area than that of the medial.

Ligaments

Because bony stability is minimal at the knee, ligaments receive a substantial amount of attention. Ligaments provide restraint to excessive motions of genu recurvatum, varus and valgus motions at the knee, anterior and posterior tibial displacement, and rotary stability. The 4 major ligaments that surround the knee are the anterior cruciate ligament (ACL), posterior cruciate ligament (PCL), medial collateral ligament (MCL), and lateral collateral ligament (LCL).

The ACL and the PCL are centered in the midline of the knee. Both are intraarticular but extra-synovial. The synovium of the knee is extensive and covers the 2 cruciate ligaments, isolating them from the synovial fluid. The ACL runs from the anterior tibia at the anterior lateral aspect of the medial intercondylar tibial spine and extends superiorly, laterally, and posteriorly to the posteromedial aspect of the lateral femoral condyle. The ACL consists of 2 bundles: an anteromedial bundle and a posterolateral bundle. The ACL limits anterior translation of the tibia on the femur. The ACL also becomes taut at the end of tibiofemoral hyperextension and during rotations of the tibia on the femur and rotation motions of the femur on the tibia.

◆ *Posterior cruciate ligament.* The PCL originates from the medial femoral condyle and descends posteriorly to insert on a ridge along the posterior tibia. The PCL functions to limit posterior translation of the tibia on the femur or anterior translation of the femur on the tibia. The PCL becomes taut at the end of extreme knee flexion. The PCL is shorter and more robust than the ACL, with a cross-sectional area approximately 120% to 150% of that of the ACL. The PCL has

Clinical Tips

Soft tissue synovial pleats inside the inner surface of the knee can become thickened and fibrotic with repetitive knee flexion and extension, creating a pathologically inflamed knee. This condition is known as plica syndrome and can cause the knee to feel stiff and have limited ROM.

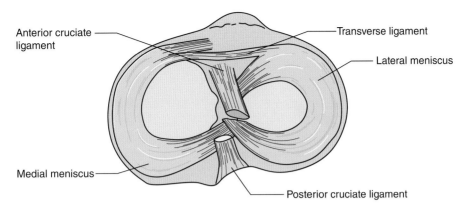

Figure 11.3 The medial and lateral meniscus provide improved joint congruence, distribute weight-bearing forces, reduce friction, and provide shock absorption.

both a posteromedial and anterolateral bundle. The respective bundles become tight or lax during knee flexion and extension movements.

◆ *Medial collateral ligament.* The MCL is a flat, broad ligament that arises superiorly from the medial femoral epicondyle and runs distally to insert onto the proximal medial tibia. The MCL has both superficial and deep portions that provide static support of the medial knee. The superficial portion attachments are described above, whereas the deep MCL portion is continuous with the medial joint capsule and is attached to the medial meniscus. Both portions restrain valgus stress placed on the tibiofemoral joint.

◆ *Lateral collateral ligament.* The LCL is more tubular in nature, running vertical from the head of the fibula in a superior direction to the lateral epicondyle of the femur. There are no attachments of the LCL to the lateral meniscus. The LCL provides a restraint to varus stress placed on the tibiofemoral joint.

Joint Kinematics

Each of the joints of the knee has a different array of movement patterns that although independent

of one another help to facilitate or hinder full movement of the other. The joint kinematics described here are due to the joint bony surfaces, interposing articular cartilage, and surrounding soft tissues.

Tibiofemoral Joint

The tibiofemoral joint has movement that occurs through 2 planes of motion. Knee flexion and extension occur around a mediolateral axis of rotation, whereas medial and lateral rotation occur around a superoinferior axis.

Arthrokinematics of the tibiofemoral joint include accessory motions of roll and glide of either the tibia on the femur (open kinetic chain) or femur on tibia (closed kinetic chain). Flexion and extension of the knee involve rolling and gliding of either component of the joint and will depend on weight-bearing status. During weight bearing (a closed chain pattern), the femur will move on the tibia, which is relatively fixed (figure 11.4*a*). During non-weight-bearing movements (open chain pattern), the tibia will move on a relatively fixed femur (figure 11.4*b*).

An excellent example of a closed kinetic chain pattern at the tibiofemoral joint is the squat

Clinical Tips

It is extremely important to fully mobilize the tibiofemoral joint to regain all knee flexion and extension range of motion. The most important motion to regain is anterior tibial glide for full knee extension mobility. If this motion is not returned, the client will ambulate with a flexed knee gait pattern, which causes patellar tendon overuse and continued pain and irritation.

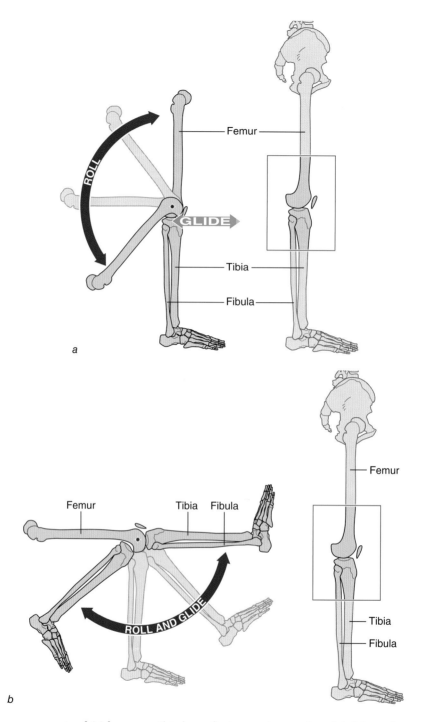

Figure 11.4 Knee movements of *(a)* femur on tibia knee flexion and extension; *(b)* tibia on femur knee flexion and extension.

exercise. During the squat, as the individual is moving from a position of full knee extension to knee flexion, the femoral condyles will move on the fixed tibia. The convex condyles of the femur will roll posteriorly on the concave tibial plateau. This could become problematic if the condyles purely rolled with no other translation, as the condyles would eventually roll off the back of the tibia. Due

to an intact ACL, as the condyles roll posteriorly, the tethering effect of the ligament helps creates an anterior slide or glide. This gliding occurs as almost a pure spinning of the condyle on the tibia. When moving from a position of knee flexion to knee extension during the squat, the femur rolls anteriorly with a simultaneous posterior glide. This occurs in part due to the restraining effect of the posterior cruciate ligament becoming taut as the condyles roll anterior. The gliding occurs as almost a pure spinning as the femur rolls anteriorly.

The tibiofemoral joint moves in motions of lateral and medial rotation when the knee is not in full extension. During motions of knee flexion and extension the tibia can laterally rotate from 0° to 20° and medially rotate from 0° to 15°. In open chain patterns, these motions occur as tibia on femur (figure 11.5a). In closed chain patterns, these motions occur as femur on tibia (figure 11.5b). These motions occur as axial rotation along a longitudinal superoinferior axis through the knee around the transverse plane. With the knee in the closed packed position there is minimal to no motion that occurs, while at 90° of

knee flexion, a maximum of about 45° of rotation occurs. Part of this motion occurs as the "screw-home mechanism." During the final degrees of open chain knee extension range of motion, an obligatory lateral rotation of the tibia occurs (figure 11.6). This automatic locking of the knee occurs because of the size of the femoral condyles and the tibial plateau. Because the medial femoral condyle is longer than the lateral, during knee extension the medial tibial plateau will continue to glide longer than that of the lateral side of the joint. This continuation of medial side movement while the lateral side has reached the end of it movement creates the obligate lateral rotation. This is most evident in the last 5° to 10° of knee extension.

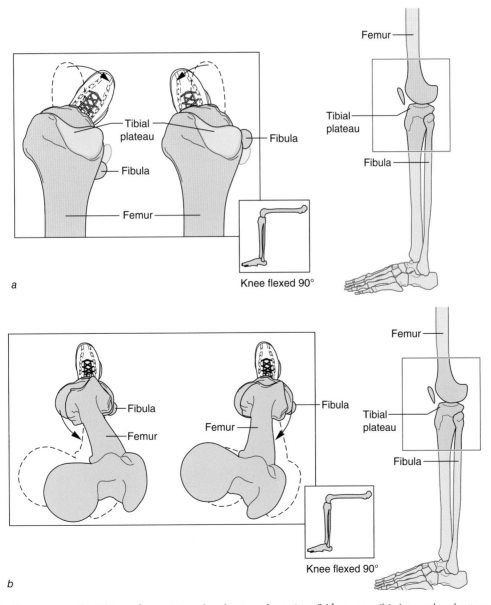

Figure 11.5 Movements of (a) tibia on femur internal and external rotation; (b) femur on tibia internal and external rotation.

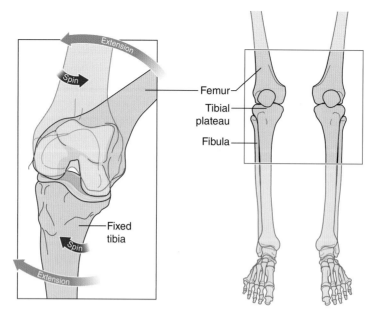

Figure 11.6 The "screw-home mechanism" of the knee.

Not considered a true motion at the knee, slight amounts of varus and valgus motion exist in the frontal plane along an anterior posterior axis. This motion is minimal to none while the knee is in full extension, and greatest when the knee is in the loose packed position.

Patellofemoral Joint

The patellofemoral joint is a modified plane joint formed by the anterior patellar trochlea of the distal femur and the posterior facets of the patella. The lateral articular surface of the patella is wider than the medial surface.

Motions are glides, tilts, and rotations. Patellar flexion and extension occur in the sagittal plane as gliding motions as the articular surface of the patella slides along the femur or of the femur sliding on the posterior surface of the patella pending the given movement (open vs. closed chain pattern) (figure 11.7). During an open kinetic chain movement pattern in which the tibia is free to move (such as kicking a soccer ball), the patella slides along the anterior femur. However, in a closed kinetic chain movement pattern (such as squatting), the patella is essentially tethered between the tibia and femur, and movement will occur as the anterior distal femur glides along the stationary patella.

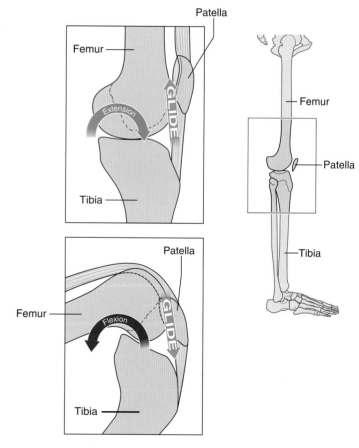

Figure 11.7 Open kinetic chain movements of the patella across the femur during knee extension and flexion.

Clinical Tips

Following any anterior knee traumatic injury or surgery, movement of the patellofemoral joint can become extremely limited. This is especially true following open surgical procedures in which the anterior knee has been incised to gain surgical exposure. Patellofemoral mobilizations are critical to gaining full knee mobility.

The patella also glides both medial and lateral as translations in the frontal plane. During lateral patellar glide, the lateral edge of the patella moves closer to the lateral femoral trochlea, whereas when gliding medial, the medial edge of the patella moves closer to the medial femoral trochlea.

Tilting of the patella occurs around a vertical axis in the transverse plane. Tilting is described by which direction the reference patellar facet is moving. During a medial patellar tilt, the medial posterior facet moves closer to the medial femoral trochlea, whereas a lateral tilt moves the lateral posterior surface of the patella closer toward the lateral trochlea.

Rotation can also occur around an anteroposterior axis along the frontal plane. A lateral patellar rotation describes a motion in which the inferior pole of the patella moves laterally from midline, while a medial rotation occurs when the inferior pole of the patella moves medially from midline. Tilting can occur in the sagittal plane along the medial/lateral axis. During an inferior patellar tilt (posterior), the inferior pole is closer to the tibial tubercle. During a superior patellar tilt (anterior), the inferior patellar pole is elevated.

KNEE JOINT ARTHROLOGY

Articular surfaces	Closed packed position	Resting position	Capsular pattern	ROM norms	End-feel
Tibiofemoral					
Tibia: inferior Femur: superior	Full extension	30° of knee flexion	Flexion > extension	0°–150°	Flexion = soft tissue Extension = firm
Patellofemoral					
Patella: posterior Femur: anterior	Full knee flexion	Full extension to 5° flexion	No true capsular pattern	Superior to inferior 11 mm	Not described

Distraction

Client position: Seated with knee extending over edge of treatment table. The tibiofemoral joint is in a resting position if a conservative technique is indicated. Clinician can adjust range for a more aggressive technique.

Clinician position: Sitting or standing at client's foot facing the involved knee. Both hands grasp the proximal tibia on both the medial and lateral sides.

Stabilization: Provided by the weight of the upper leg and pelvis on the treatment table.

Mobilization: Both hands simultaneously distract the tibia distally in a direction parallel to the long axis of the tibia.

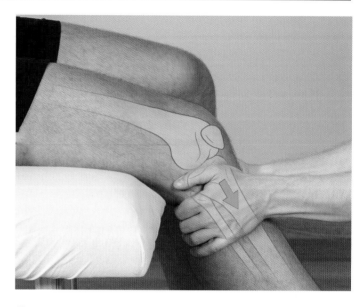

Goal of technique: To increase general overall mobility of the tibiofemoral joint.

Note: This technique does not benefit a particular knee movement but is an excellent mobilization for overall mobility.

Dorsal Glide of Tibia on Femur

Client position: Either supine or sitting, depending on whether using a conservative or an aggressive technique, or based on clinician preference.

Clinician position: Sitting at client's foot facing the involved knee.

Stabilization: Proximal hand can be used to support the femur if client is supine; if client is sitting over edge of table, proximal hand can be used to help mobilize.

Mobilization: The manipulating hand grasps the proximal tibia from the ventral side and glides the tibia in a dorsal direction.

Goal of technique: To increase knee flexion mobility.

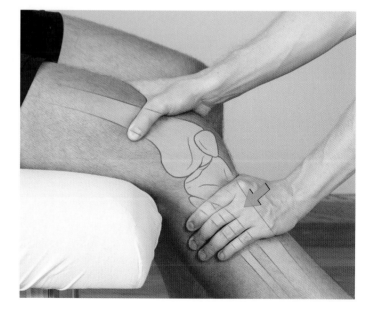

Notes: This is an excellent mobilization to increase knee flexion. The clinician might choose to add internal rotation to this technique.

Ventral Glide of Tibia on Femur 1

Client position: Supine, with knee in resting position if a conservative technique is used, approximating end range if a more aggressive technique is used.

Clinician position: Standing alongside client's knee.

Stabilization: Proximal hand holds the femur; distal mobilizing hand grasps the tibia.

Mobilization: Distal mobilizing hand glides the tibia in the ventral direction. If knee is in a greater degree of flexion, both hands can be used to glide the tibia in a ventral direction.

Goal of technique: To increase knee extension mobility.

Notes: This technique is great for knee extension range of motion. It might be beneficial to add an external rotation force onto tibia.

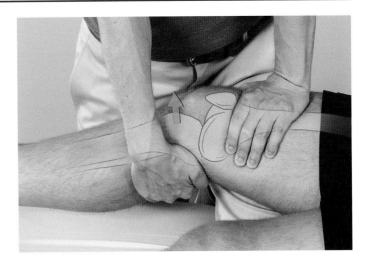

Ventral Glide of Tibia on Femur 2

VIDEO 11.1 **in the web study guide shows this technique.**

Client position: Supine, with knee approximating full extension.

Clinician position: Standing alongside client on the side of the involved knee. Clinician places 1 or both hands on top of the ventral surface of the distal femur.

Stabilization: Place a pillow or towel under the proximal tibia.

Mobilization: Femur is mobilized in a dorsal direction, thus producing a "relative" ventral glide of the tibia on the femur.

Goal of technique: To increase knee extension mobility.

Note: This is a great technique when pressure through tibia is contraindicated for any reason.

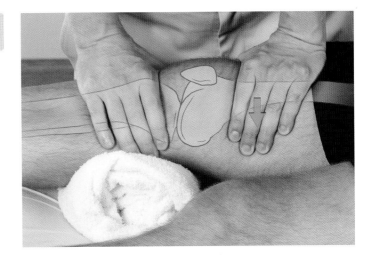

Ventral Glide of Tibia on Femur 3

Client position: Prone, with knee approximating full extension. A towel or pillow is placed at the anterior aspect of the client's foot/ankle.

Clinician position: Standing alongside client on side of involved knee.

Stabilization: The stabilizing hand maintains the distal leg on the towel roll. The thigh is stabilized by bodyweight.

Mobilization: The manipulating hand is placed over the dorsal surface of the proximal tibia and glides it in a ventral direction.

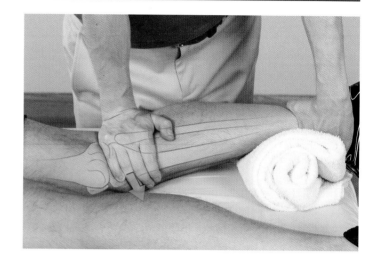

Goal of technique: To increase knee extension mobility.

Note: This is a good mobilization that allows great patient relaxation because of the support from the table.

Medial Glide

Client position: Either supine or sitting in a resting position if a conservative technique is used, approximating end range of restriction if a more aggressive technique is used.

Clinician position: Standing alongside involved extremity, or seated at end of table between client's knees. Client's lower leg is held between clinician's arm and trunk.

Stabilization: Proximal hand grasps and holds the distal femur from the medial side.

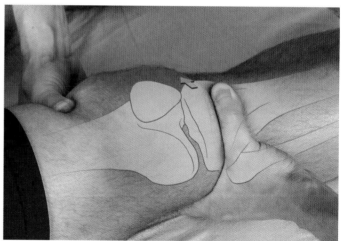

Mobilization: Distal manipulating hand gasps the proximal tibia and fibula from the lateral side and glides the proximal tibia in a medial direction indirectly through the fibula.

Lateral Glide

Client position: Supine or sitting. Resting position if a conservative technique is used, approximating end range of restriction if a more aggressive technique is used.

Clinician position: Seated on edge of table, or standing alongside involved extremity. Client's lower leg is held between clinician's arm and trunk.

Stabilization: Proximal stabilizing hand grasps and holds the distal femur from the lateral side.

Mobilization: Distal manipulating hand grasps the proximal tibia from the medial side and glides the proximal tibia in a lateral direction while the trunk guides this motion.

Goal of technique: To increase overall tibiofemoral mobility.

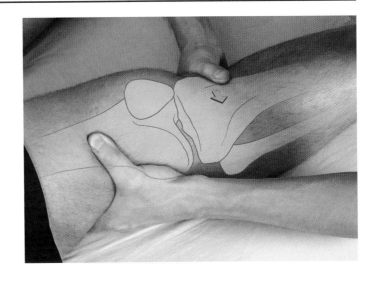

Medial Gap

Client position: Either supine or sitting. Resting position if a conservative technique is used, approximating end range of restriction if a more aggressive technique is used.

Clinician position: At foot of treatment table facing client's knee, with client's lower leg between clinician's arm and trunk.

Stabilization: Distal hand supports the distal lower leg from the medial side while holding the foot and ankle against the trunk.

Mobilization: Proximal hand grasps the lateral side of the knee at the joint line and moves the knee medially at the lateral joint line, gapping the medial side of the joint.

Goal of technique: To increase overall tibiofemoral mobility.

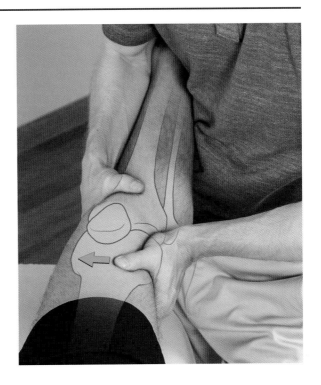

Lateral Gap

Client position: Either supine or sitting. Resting position if a conservative technique is used, approximating end range of restriction if a more aggressive technique is used.

Clinician position: Standing near foot of treatment table facing client's knee, with client's lower leg between clinician's arm and trunk.

Stabilization: Distal hand supports the distal lower leg from the lateral side while holding the foot and ankle against the trunk.

Mobilization: Proximal hand grasps the medial side of the knee at the joint line and moves the knee laterally at the medial joint line, gapping the lateral side of the joint.

Goal of technique: To increase overall tibiofemoral mobility.

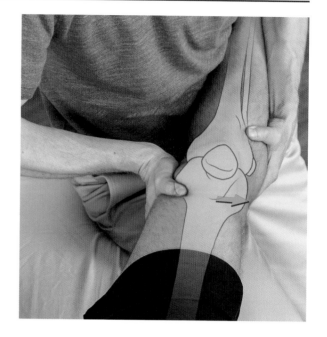

PFJ Cranial Glide

VIDEO 11.2 **in the web study guide shows this technique.**

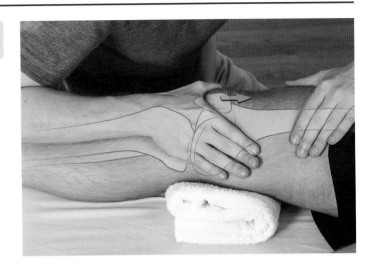

Client position: Supine with a towel roll placed under knee for comfort and to maintain slight knee flexion.

Clinician position: Sitting alongside involved knee facing the patellofemoral joint.

Stabilization: Cranial hand stabilizes the femur.

Mobilization: Distal hand is positioned with web space on caudal surface of patella. Ensure the forearm is along the tibia. The manipulating hand glides the patella cranially.

Goal of technique: To increase knee extension mobility.

Note: Mobilizing from a plane that is not parallel to the patellofemoral joint can cause irritation from compression of the infrapatellar fat pad.

PFJ Caudal Glide

Client position: Supine with a towel roll placed under knee for comfort and to maintain slight knee flexion.

Clinician Position: Sitting alongside client's hip facing distally toward the patellofemoral joint.

Stabilization: Caudal hand stabilizes the lower leg.

Mobilization: Proximal hand is positioned with web space on cranial surface of patella. Ensure forearm is along femur. The manipulating hand glides patella caudally, ensuring not to compress patella into femur.

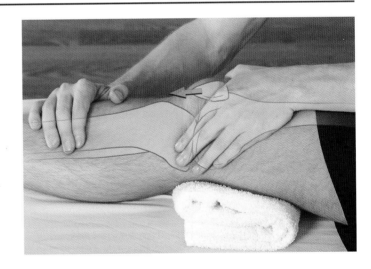

Goal of technique: To increase knee flexion mobility.

Note: Mobilizing from a plane that is not parallel to the patellofemoral joint can cause irritation from compression of the superior joint capsule.

PFJ Medial Glide

 VIDEO 11.3 in the web study guide shows this technique.

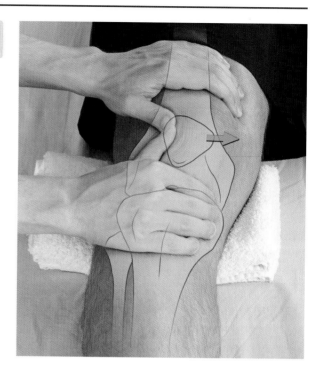

Client position: Supine with a towel roll placed under knee for comfort and to maintain slight flexion.

Clinician position: Sitting alongside client's knee, facing affected patellofemoral joint. Both hands are positioned with either the thumbs or the heel of one hand on the lateral surface of the patella.

Stabilization: Free hand/fingers stabilize the lower extremity, preventing rotation.

Mobilization: The heel of the hand or both thumbs glide the patella in a medial direction.

Goal of technique: To increase overall patellofemoral mobility by stretching lateral superficial retinaculum.

PFJ Lateral Glide

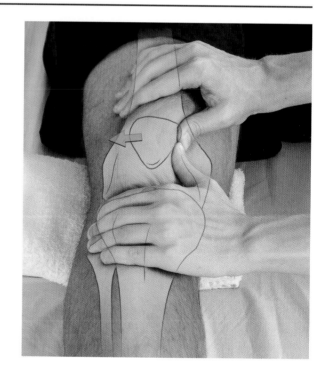

Client position: Supine with a towel roll placed under knee for comfort and to maintain slight flexion.

Clinician position: Sitting alongside client's knee, facing affected patellofemoral joint. Both hands are positioned with either the thumbs of both or the heel of one hand on the medial surface of the patella.

Stabilization: Free hand/fingers stabilize the lower extremity, preventing rotation.

Mobilization: The heel of the hand or both thumbs glides the patella in a lateral direction.

Goal of technique: To increase overall patellofemoral mobility by stretching medial superficial retinaculum.

PFJ Medial Tilt

VIDEO 11.4 **in the web study guide shows this technique.**

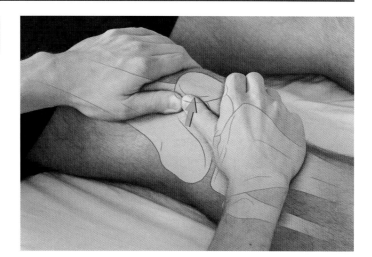

Client position: Supine with knee in full extension.

Clinician position: Sitting alongside client's knee facing affected patellofemoral joint. Both hands are positioned with both thumbs under the inferior lateral edge of the patella.

Stabilization: Index fingers prevent the patella from sliding medially.

Mobilization: The thumbs simultaneously tilt the patella in a medial direction.

Goal of technique: To increase overall patellofemoral mobility by stretching lateral deep retinaculum.

PFJ Lateral Tilt

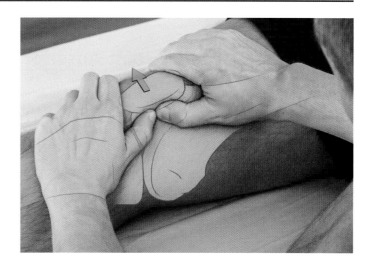

Client position: Supine with the knee in full extension.

Clinician position: Sitting alongside client's knee facing affected patellofemoral joint. Hands are positioned with both thumbs under the inferior lateral edge of the patella.

Stabilization: Index fingers prevent the patella from sliding laterally.

Mobilization: The thumbs simultaneously tilt the patella in a lateral direction.

Goal of technique: To increase overall patellofemoral mobility by stretching the medial deep retinaculum.

Proximal Tibiofibular Joint Posterior Glide

Client position: Supine with knee slightly flexed.

Clinician position: Standing facing client on side to be assessed.

Stabilization: Clinician's hand purchases medial proximal tibia.

Mobilization: Heel of clinician's assessing hand purchases anterior surface of fibular head and glides fibula in a posterior direction along plane of joint.

Goal of technique: Adjust a ventral positional fault of the proximal fibula.

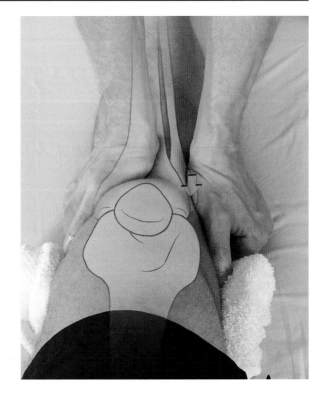

Proximal Tibiofibular Joint Anterior Glide

Client position: Prone with knee slightly flexed.

Clinician position: Standing on side to be assessed.

Stabilization: Clinician's hand purchases medial proximal tibia.

Mobilization: Heel of clinician's hand purchases posterior surface of fibular head and glides fibula in an anterior direction along plane of joint.

Goal of technique: Adjust a dorsal position fault of the proximal fibula.

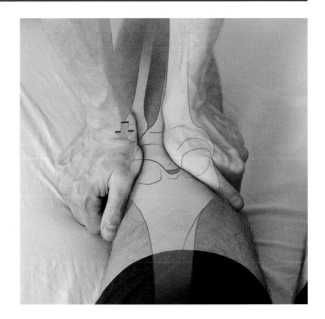

Go to the web study guide and complete the case study for this chapter. The case study discusses a 24-year-old male with ACL and MCL injuries following a motorcycle accident.

EVIDENCE FOR MANUAL THERAPY OF VARIOUS KNEE JOINT PATHOLOGIES

Study	Clients	Intervention and comparison (if any)	Outcome(s)
Utilization of thrust and nonthrust mobilization for anterior cruciate ligament reconstruction: Grade C			
Hunt et al., 2010 (Level 3)	12 patients with knee extension ROM deficits following ACL reconstruction	Single session of anterior tibiofemoral glides on knee extension in those with knee extension deficits following anterior cruciate ligament reconstruction	Single session of anterior tibiofemoral glides increases maximal knee extension in those with knee extension deficits. These increases were small and short lived.
Utilization of thrust and nonthrust mobilization and manipulation for knee osteoarthritis: Grade C			
Deyle et al., 2005 (Level 1)	154 subjects with knee osteoarthritis	Compared home-based treatment versus clinic-based treatment, which included individualized manual therapy including joint mobilizations	Clinical treatment group that included joint mobilizations to knee achieved twice as much improvement in WOMAC scores than unsupervised.
Silvernail et al., 2011 (Level 3)	20 subjects with symptomatic knee osteoarthritis	Therapist applied joint mobilizations in 2 grades (III and IV) while capacitance-based pressure mat captured characteristics of force and frequency. Reliability measures were also determined.	Force measurements for grade III in extension were 45,74N; for flexion were 39,61N; for medial/lateral glide were 20,34N; for inferior glide were 18,35N. Force measurements for grade IV in extension were 57,76N; for flexion were 47,68N; for medial/lateral glides were 23,36N; for inferior glides were 18,35N. Inter-class correlation coefficients were above 0.90 for almost all measures.
Deyle et al., 2012 (Level 3)	120 patients with knee osteoarthritis	Extracted data from standardized examination forms to determine predictors of nonsuccess	Patellofemoral pain, anterior cruciate ligament laxity and height > 1.71 m comprise the CPR. Patients with at least 2 positive tests yielded a posttest probability of 88% for nonsuccess with this treatment.
Abbott et al., 2013 (Level 1)	206 adults with hip or knee osteoarthritis	Randomly allocated to receive: (1) manual therapy, (2) multimodal exercise, (3) combined exercise and manual therapy, (4) no therapy	Manual therapy provided benefits over usual care that were sustained to 1 year.

ROM = range of motion; ACL = anterior cruciate ligament; WOMAC = Western Ontario and McMaster Universities Arthritis Index; N = Newtons; CPR = clinical prediction rule

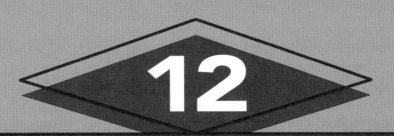

ANKLE JOINT

LEARNING OBJECTIVES

After completing this chapter, you will be able to do the following:

- Describe the bony and soft tissue anatomy of the ankle complex
- Describe the joint kinematics of the ankle joint
- Describe appropriate positioning, movements, and intentions for ankle joint mobilization techniques
- Identify evidence supporting ankle joint mobilization techniques

The ankle joint complex consists of a stable syndesmotic distal tibiofibular joint and a relatively simple talocrural joint. Movement at these joints is imperative for functional maneuvers such as walking, running, and jumping. Limited movement in this complex will cause compensation above at the knee or below at the subtalar joint.

Ankle sprains are one of the most common injuries of the lower leg. Inappropriate treatment and rehabilitation can result in residual symptoms, recurrent ankle injuries, and ultimately chronic ankle instability. Assessment and treatment of faulty joint motion is critical in returning the ankle mechanics back to normal.

Anatomy

The ankle joint complex consists of the distal tibiofibular joint and the talocrural joint. These articulations are important for absorbing and distributing ground reaction forces. They also help transmit energy from the foot to the lower leg.

Distal Tibiofibular Joint

The distal tibiofibular joint consists of the distal tibia and fibula and forms a "roof" over the talus (figure 12.1). This articulation is classified as a synarthrodial syndesmosis and adds to the stability of the ankle joint. The surfaces of the tibia and fibula are flat, oval facets covered with cartilage and connected by an articular capsule and by the anterior tibiofibular ligament and the posterior tibiofibular ligament. Additionally, the crural interosseous tibiofibular ligament connects the tibia and fibula and is continuous with the interosseous membrane. These soft tissue structures constitute the chief bond of union between the tibia and fibula and provide stability for the mortise of the ankle joint.

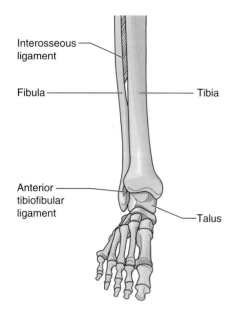

Figure 12.1 Distal tibiofibular joint.

Talocrural Joint

The talocrural joint is the true "ankle" joint consisting of the distal tibia (tibial plafond) and fibula (medial/lateral malleolus) and the trochlea of the talus. This joint is classified as a uniaxial hinge joint. The concave distal tibiofibular joint articulates with the convex talar dome. The stability of the joint is provided by ligaments medially (deltoid ligament) and laterally (anterior talofibular, posterior talofibular, calcaneofibular ligaments) (figure 12.2). The deltoid ligament has two layers: a superficial and a deep. The superficial layer consists of the tibionavicular, tibiocalcaneal, and posterior tibiotalar ligaments. The tibionavicular ligament runs from the medial malleolus to the navicular bone and spring ligament. The tibiocalcaneal ligament runs from the medial malleolus to the sustentaculum tali. The posterior tibiotalar ligament attaches from the medial malleolus to the posterior talus process. The deep layer is the anterior tibiotalar ligament, which travels from the medial malleolus to the navicular bone. The strong deltoid ligament helps to stabilize the medial ankle and prevent excessive eversion, external rotation, and plantarflexion. The anterior talofibular ligament and the posterior talofibular ligament provide support to the talocrural joint. The anterior ligament is under greater tension in plantarflexion. The calcaneofibular ligament plays an important role in providing stability to both the talocrural and the subtalar joints. The calcaneofibular ligament is under greater tension in ankle dorsiflexion.

The posterior joint is covered by the Achilles tendon (figure 12.3). The Achilles tendon is the strongest tendon in the human body and provides exceptional recoil ability to propel the body forward during running and jumping. It has also been suggested that tightness in the talocrural joint may lead to Achilles tendinitis (Irwin, 2014).

Joint Kinematics

The joint kinematics of the distal tibiofibular joint and talocrural joint are fairly straightforward. These two joints work in synchrony such that motion at the talocrural joint is accompanied by conjunct motion at the distal tibiofibular joint. The clinician must examine both joints when assessing ankle motion.

Distal Tibiofibular Joint

Because of the nature of the joint, the distal tibiofibular joint has very little motion. The talus is wider anteriorly than posteriorly and therefore a small amount of mortise separation (1–3 mm) occurs with dorsiflexion. The fibula rotates laterally (2°–3°) and glides proximally (superior) to allow for the movement of the talus into the mortise. During plantarflexion, the fibula rotates medially, which narrows the mortise, and subsequently the talus moves out of the mortise. Weight-bearing motion at the talocrural and subtalar joint influences motion of the tibia. Pronation and dorsiflexion is accompanied by internal rotation of the tibia.

Talocrural Joint

The talocrural joint has motion that occurs primarily in the sagittal plane about a medial to lateral axis. Specifically, the axis of the talocrural joint runs just distal to both the medial and lateral malleoli. In the transverse plane, the axis deviates approximately 10° to 20° from the medial to lateral axis (figure 12.4).

In open chain dorsiflexion, the talus rolls anteriorly and glides posteriorly and abducts on the tibia as it moves into the mortise (figure 12.5). During dorsiflexion, the calcaneofibular ligament and posterior capsule become taut. The motion of plantarflexion is opposite of dorsiflexion, with the talus rolling posteriorly and sliding anteriorly. The anterior talofibular ligament, tibionavicular ligament, and anterior capsule become taut with plantarflexion.

The weight-bearing dorsiflexion arthrokinematics are the same as the non-weight-bearing ones, although the motion is more dramatic and usually described by the proximal segment. With weight-bearing dorsiflexion, the distal tibia and fibula glide anteriorly on a relatively fixed talus.

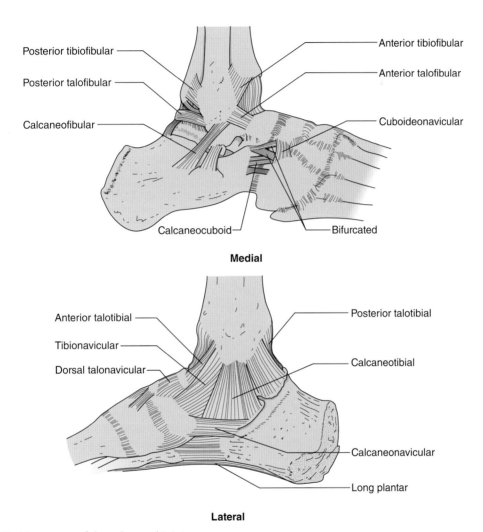

Figure 12.2 Ligaments of the talocrural joint.

Clinical Tips

A high ankle sprain is an injury to the interosseous membrane (syndesmosis) and anterior tibiofibular ligament that occurs secondary to twisting of the tibia inward while the foot is dorsiflexed and everted. This type of sprain is more common in sports such as football and soccer. Healing of this type of sprain is tricky because of the stress placed on the injured structures during weight-bearing activity such as walking (Hoch and McKeon, 2010).

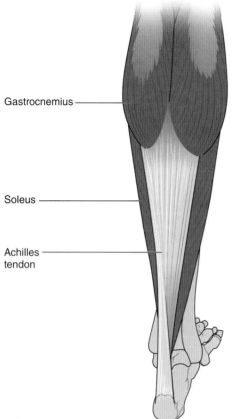

Figure 12.3 Achilles tendon.

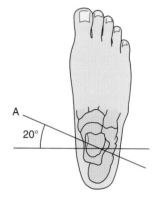

Figure 12.4 Axis of the talocrural joint.

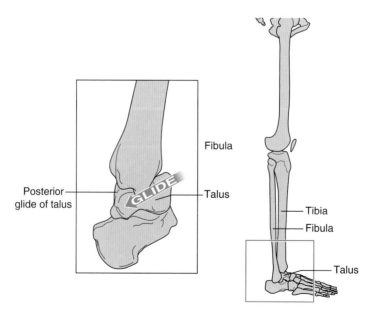

Figure 12.5 Open chain arthrokinematics of dorsiflexion.

This motion is more pronounced in the tibia on the talus, resulting in internal rotation of tibia (figure 12.6). Weight-bearing plantarflexion will result in a heel raise maneuver. During weight-bearing plantarflexion, the fibula glides posteriorly more profoundly than the tibia on the talus, resulting in external rotation of the tibia, and the talus slides anteriorly and laterally.

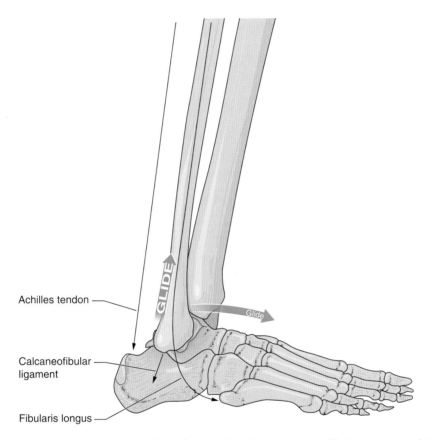

Figure 12.6 Closed chain arthrokinematics of dorsiflexion. Weight-bearing dorsiflexion consists of the tibia and fibula gliding anteriorly over the fixed talus. The fibula conjunctly superiorly glides and internally rotates.

ANKLE JOINT ARTHROLOGY

Articular surfaces	Closed packed position	Resting position	Capsular pattern	ROM norms	End-feel
Distal tibiofibular joint					
Convex lower end of fibula and the concave fibular notch of the distal tibia	Not applicable	Not applicable	Pain when joint stressed	No active range of motion	Not applicable
Talocrural joint					
OKC Moving surface is talus (convex); stable surface is distal tibia and fibula (concave) **CKC** Moving surface is distal tibia and fibula (concave) moving on stationary talus (convex)	Maximum dorsiflexion	10° of plantarflexion, midway between inversion and eversion	Plantarflexion limited more than dorsiflexion	Dorsiflexion: 20° Plantarflexion: 50°	Firm for dorsiflexion and plantarflexion; plantarflexion can be hard if posterior tubercle of talus contacts posterior tibia

OKC = open kinetic chain; CKC = closed kinetic chain

Anterior Glide

Client position: Side-lying with medial border of foot on treatment table.

Clinician position: Standing behind client facing heel of foot to be treated.

Stabilization: Clinician's cranial hand stabilizes the distal tibia.

Mobilization: Clinician's thumbs are placed along the posterior shelf of the distal fibula. Clinician applies an anteriorly directed force on the distal fibula. (The thenar eminence can be used in place of thumb at clinician's discretion.)

Goal of technique: To achieve restricted motion of the talocrural joint.

Note: This technique can also be performed with the client in a prone position or with the fibula stabilized and the tibia glided.

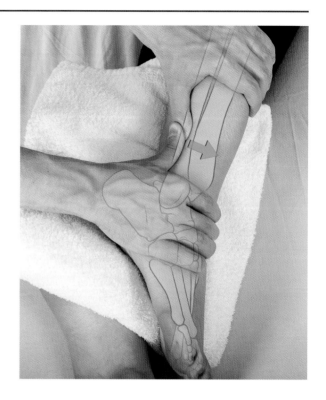

Posterior Glide

 VIDEO 12.1 **in the web study guide shows this technique.**

Client position: Supine with foot resting on treatment table.

Clinician position: Standing at foot of treatment table facing client's foot.

Stabilization: Clinician's inside hand stabilizes the distal tibia against the treatment table.

Mobilization: Clinician applies a posteriorly directed force using the thenar eminence of the outside hand on the distal fibula.

Goal of technique: To improve motion associated with restriction of talocrural joint.

Note: This technique can also be performed with the client in a side-lying position or with the fibula stabilized and the tibia glided.

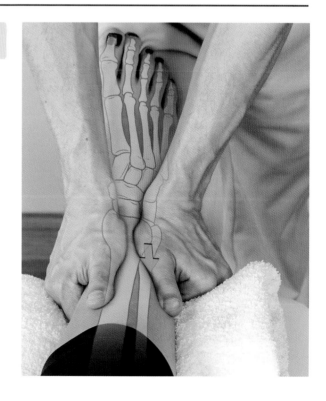

Weight-Bearing Anterior Glide of the Fibula

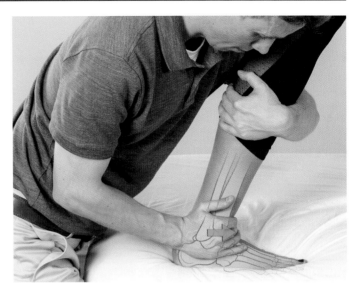

Client position: Standing on treatment table with nontreated leg in front to widen base of support.

Clinician position: Standing behind client on the ground.

Stabilization: Clinician's nonmobilizing hand wraps around the entire lower limb and grasps the posterior calf.

Mobilization: Clinician's mobilizing hand is perched on the distal fibula. This hand applies an anterior glide to the fibula. Once end range is reached with the glide, a minimal internal rotation spin is performed to the lower leg.

Goals of technique: To increase mobility in the lateral capsule of the talocrural joint and facilitate internal rotation of the lower limb that accompanies dorsiflexion.

Note: A mobilization wedge can be used under the medial side of the foot.

Superior Glide of Fibula

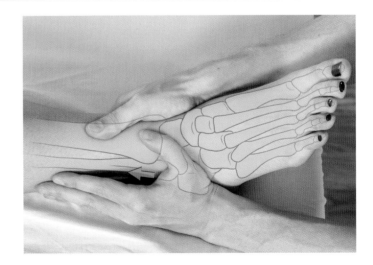

Client position: Supine with foot relaxed on treatment table.

Clinician position: Seated at foot of treatment table facing client.

Stabilization: Clinician's nonmobilizing hand grasps the distal tibia with a firm hand hold. Client's leg on treatment table adds stability.

Mobilization: Clinician uses the thenar eminence purchased under the distal fibula of client. A superiorly directed force is applied to the fibula.

Goal of technique: To achieve full dorsiflexion of the talocrural joint, the fibula glides superiorly.

Note: Material such as Theraband can be used to prevent slipping of the contact hand.

Inferior Glide of Fibula

Client position: Side-lying with mobilizing foot on top and supported with a folded towel.

Clinician position: Standing or sitting facing back of client's leg.

Stabilization: Clinician's proximal hand grasps the distal fibula using a pincer grasp. The clinician's distal hand grasps the hindfoot. Table contact provides stabilization.

Mobilization: A caudal glide of the fibula is performed by the clinician, inverting the hindfoot and applying a slight inferior pressure on the distal fibula.

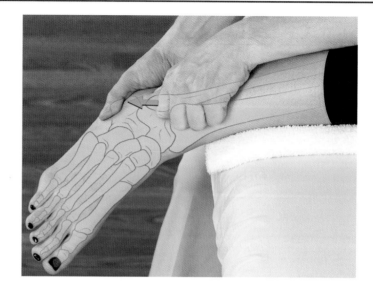

Goal of technique: To achieve limited talocrural motion.

Note: Material such as Theraband can be used to prevent slipping of the contact hand.

Distraction

Client position: Supine with talocrural joint in resting position.

Clinician position: Sitting with medial to lower leg facing dorsal aspect of client's foot.

Stabilization: Clinician cradles foot using both hands, one on top of ankle and the other on the posterior side of ankle.

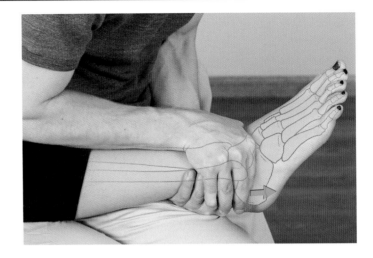

Mobilization: Clinician's anterior hand grasps as close to the joint as possible around the anterior talus. The posterior hand grasps the posterior talus directly proximal to the posterior calcaneus. With forearms in line with long axis of lower leg, clinician leans away from client's head, distracting the talus distally.

Goal of technique: To increase overall range of motion.

Notes: Clinician may cradle the lower leg and ankle next to his or her trunk. This technique may be less appropriate for a client with pathological problems with ligamentous restraint to the hip or knee.

Distraction Thrust

VIDEO 12.2 in the web study guide shows this technique.

Client position: Supine with involved foot over edge of treatment table.

Clinician position: Facing client at foot of treatment table.

Stabilization: Clinician grasps dorsum of foot with interlaced fingers. Clinician's thumbs rest on the plantar surface of client's foot.

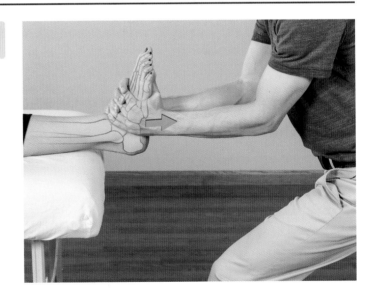

Mobilization: Clinician applies a high-velocity, low-amplitude thrust to the talocrural joint by leaning backward and shifting weight to back leg.

Goal of technique: To improve dorsiflexion range of motion following an ankle sprain.

Note: This same setup can be used for mobilization techniques.

Posterior Talar Glide

 VIDEO 12.3 in the web study guide shows this technique.

Client position: Supine with talocrural joint in resting position and the foot over the edge of the treatment table.

Clinician position: Standing at end of treatment table facing dorsal surface of foot.

Stabilization: Clinician's stabilizing hand maintains position on the distal posterior surface of the lower leg, holding leg in place.

Mobilization: Clinician's mobilizing hand grips anterior surface of the talus and glides it in a posterior direction.

Goal of technique: To increase ankle dorsiflexion.

Note: This technique can also be performed with the stabilizing hand on the anterior surface of the tibia.

Clinical tips: 95% of all ankle sprains are lateral. A lateral ankle sprain is injury to the lateral ligaments of the ankle, most commonly the anterior talofibular ligament. The mechanism of injury is forced inversion and plantarflexion. Following a lateral ankle sprain, the position of the talus may remain anterior, causing an anterior impingement of the talus with tibial plafond (Denegar, Hertel, and Fonseca, 2002). Individuals may describe anterior joint pain when trying to increase dorsiflexion, for instance with gastrosoleus stretching. The posterior talar glide is a good technique to help correct anterior positional fault of the talus.

Posterior Talar Glide: Weight-Bearing Mobilization With Movement

Client position: Standing with involved foot on a step-stool in front or on a treatment table that can be elevated.

Clinician position: Standing in walk-stance position facing client.

Stabilization: A mobilization belt is placed around client's upper ankle and clinician's hips.

Mobilization: Using a double web spaced grasp over anterior aspect of client's talus, clinician applies a posteriorly directed force to the talus. Client moves into dorsiflexion at the same time as the posterior glide is applied.

Goal of technique: To improve dorsiflexion range of motion.

Posterior Talar Glide: Mobilization With Movement

Client position: Supine with foot off treatment table.

Clinician position: Standing at end of treatment table facing client. The plantar surface of client's foot is placed on clinician's thigh.

Stabilization: Clinician's nonmobilizing hand grasps the distal tibia.

Mobilization: Clinician's mobilizing hand grips anterior surface of the talus and glides it in a posterior direction. At the same time, clinician applies a dorsiflexion force to ankle by stepping in toward treatment table.

Goal of technique: To improve dorsiflexion range of motion.

Notes: The client can use a towel around the foot and pull it to impart a dorsiflexion motion.

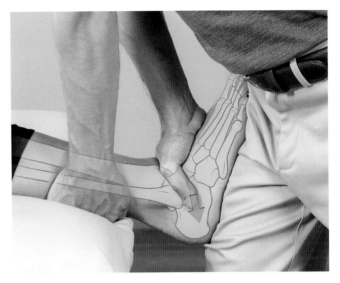

Anterior Talar Glide

Client position: Prone with talocrural joint in resting position and remainder of leg supported by treatment table.

Clinician position: Standing at end of treatment table facing posterior surface of client's lower leg.

Stabilization: Clinician's nonmobilizing hand is positioned on anterior surface of lower leg to stabilize limb.

Mobilization: If ankle is in resting position, clinician's mobilizing hand grips the talus at the posterior surface of the lower leg. If foot is in plantarflexion, mobilization can be performed through the calcaneus. The mobilizing hand glides the talus in an anterior direction.

Goal of technique: To increase plantarflexion.

Note: This technique can also be performed with the stabilizing hand on the posterior surface of the distal tibia.

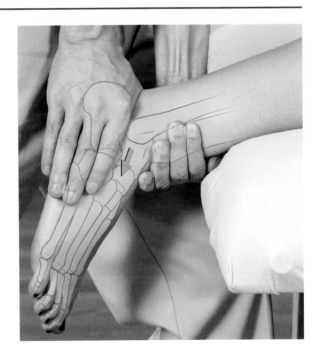

Indirect Anterior Talar Glide

Client position: Supine with talocrural joint in resting position.

Clinician position: Standing at foot of treatment table facing client's foot.

Stabilization: Clinician's stabilizing hand grips talus on posterior aspect of lower leg, holding talus in position.

Mobilization: The clinician's anterior mobilizing hand grips the distal tibia and fibula on the dorsal surface of the lower leg. The hand glides the tibia and fibula in a posterior direction, thus imparting a relative anterior force to the talus on the tibia and fibula.

Goal of Technique: To increase plantarflexion.

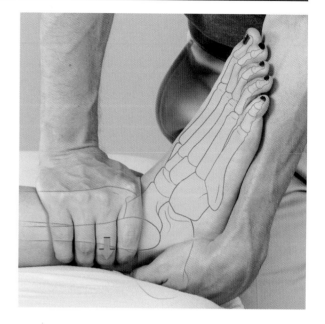

Go to the web study guide and complete the case study for this chapter. The case study discusses a 23-year-old male with lateral ankle pain after twisting his ankle.

EVIDENCE FOR MANUAL THERAPY OF VARIOUS ANKLE PATHOLOGIES

Study	Clients	Intervention and comparison (if any)	Outcome(s)
Utilization of thrust and nonthrust mobilization for chronic ankle instability: Grade A			
Cruz-Diaz et al., 2015 (Level 1b)	90 clients with recurrent ankle sprains and limited dorsiflexion	Clients were randomly assigned to Intervention, Sham Group, or Control Group; intervention was MWM technique applied 2 times a week for 3 weeks	MWM is a valuable tool to restore ankle function (ROM, dynamic postural control, self-report of instability).
Loudon et al., 2014 (Level 2a)	5 studies reviewed MT on subacute/chronic ankle sprains (134 clients)	Various MT techniques (talar AP, MWM, thrust manipulation) vs. self-control or control groups	Overall recommendation from study: MT was beneficial for improving ROM and function and diminishing pain.
Vicenzino et al., 2006 (Level 3b)	16 clients with recurrent ankle sprain; randomized, double-blind, repeated-measures, crossover control design	Closed chain or open chain MWM vs. self-control group in crossover design	Both WB and NWB MWM improved posterior talar glide (55%, 50%) and dorsiflexion for short-term follow-up.
Utilization of thrust and nonthrust mobilization for acute ankle sprain: Grade B			
Loudon et al., 2014 (Level 2a)	3 studies reviewed MT on acute ankle sprains (110 clients)	MT and standard of care vs. standard of care in control group	Overall recommendation from study: MT was beneficial for improving ROM and diminishing pain.
Whitman et al., 2009 (Level 2b)	85 clients with acute inversion ankle sprain	Thrust and nonthrust MT to all clients	Positive short-term outcome with manipulation when 3 of 4 variables included: symptoms while standing, symptoms worse in evening, NDT ≤5mm, distal tib-fib joint hypermobile; diminish pain and improve dorsiflexion.
Utilization of thrust and nonthrust mobilization for ankle immobilization: Grade C			
Landrum et al., 2008 (Level 3b)	10 subjects with minimum of 14 days of immobilization; crossover design	Grade III posterior to anterior mobilization of talus performed followed by assessment of dorsiflexion ROM, posterior ankle joint stiffness, and posterior talar translation to immobilized ankle compared to contralateral ankle	Increased dorsiflexion ROM.

MWM = mobilization with movement, ROM = range of motion, MT = manual therapy, NDT = navicular drop test; WB = weight-bearing; NWB = non-weight-bearing; AP = anterior-posterior

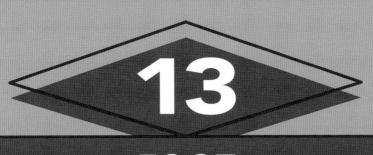

FOOT

LEARNING OBJECTIVES

After completing this chapter, you will be able to do the following:

◆ Describe the bony and soft tissue anatomy of the foot complex

◆ Describe the joint kinematics of the foot joint complex

◆ Describe appropriate positioning, movements, and intentions for the foot joint complex mobilization techniques

◆ Identify evidence supporting foot joint complex mobilization techniques

The ankle and foot contain 26 bones (14 phalanges, 5 metatarsals, 7 tarsals) plus 2 sesamoid bones (figure 13.1). This results in 33 joints with more than 100 muscles and ligaments. The joints presented in this chapter are the subtalar joint, midtarsal joints, tarsometatarsal joints, metatarsophalangeal joints, and interphalangeal joints.

These multiple joints must work in unison to complete complex tasks. For example, the foot serves as a shock absorber in the early phases of gait but switches to a rigid lever for push-off right before the foot leaves the ground. As to be expected, injuries to the foot have a devastating effect on lower extremity function. Common injuries in this area involve fractures, tendon and ligamentous injuries, and nerve entrapments.

Anatomy

The foot is a complex comprised of multiple bones and synovial joints. It can be divided into the rearfoot, midfoot, and forefoot. The rearfoot consists of the subtalar joint; the midfoot consists of the midtarsal joint; the forefoot consists of the tarsometatarsal joints, metatarsophalangeal joints, and proximal/distal interphalangeal joints.

Subtalar Joint

The subtalar joint is the articulation between the distal talus and the proximal calcaneus. This joint is a diarthrodial bicondylar joint. The superior surface of the calcaneus has 3

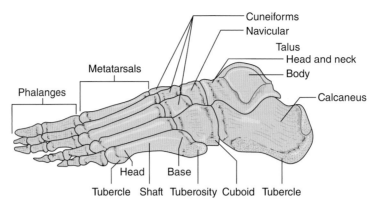

Figure 13.1 Bones of the foot.

articulating facets—a posterior, middle, and anterior facet. The posterior facet is located on the posterolateral part of the calcaneus with a convexity anterior to posterior and concavity medial/lateral. The anterior facet extends along the superomedial aspect of the calcaneus and is biconcave. The middle facet is concave and articulates with the middle calcaneal articular surface of the talus. The anterior and posterior portion of the joint is separated by the sinus tarsi. Stability of the subtalar joint is provided by the plantar calcaneonavicular ligament and the short and long plantar ligaments.

Midtarsal Joint

The midtarsal joint consists of 2 primary articulations between the calcaneocuboid joint and the talonavicular joint (figure 13.2). The calcaneocuboid joint is formed from the anterior "trumpet-like" projection of the calcaneus and posterior cuboid. This joint is classified as a saddle joint. The posterior cuboid is convex in a medial and lateral direction, and concave in a superior to inferior direction. The articulating calcaneus is just opposite.

The talonavicular joint is a condyloid synovial joint. The anterior rounded talar head articulates with the concave facet of the posterior navicular. These articulations are supported by numerous ligaments, including the plantar calcaneonavicular (spring) ligament, bifurcated (Y) ligament, and the long and short plantar ligaments.

Tarsometatarsal Joints

The tarsometatarsal joints consist of the proximal tarsal bones and the distal metatarsals. The met-

atarsals are 5 bones numbered from the medial side (figure 13.3). All 5 bones have a prismoid body that is curved longitudinally, concave inferiorly, and slightly convex superiorly. The first metatarsal is the shortest. Its body is thick and strong. The plantar surface of the head has 2 grooved facets for the sesamoid bones. The base of the first metatarsal articulates with the medial cuneiform. The second metatarsal is the longest and articulates with all cuneiforms and the base of the third metatarsal. The third articulates with third cuneiform and the second and fourth metatarsals. The fourth articulates with the cuboid, third cuneiform, and third and fifth metatarsals. The fifth articulates with the cuboid and the fourth metatarsal. The fifth metatarsal has several soft tissue attachments. The peroneus tertius (medial) and peroneus brevis (lateral) both attach to the fifth metatarsal base. The tarsometatarsal joints are diarthrodial plane joints.

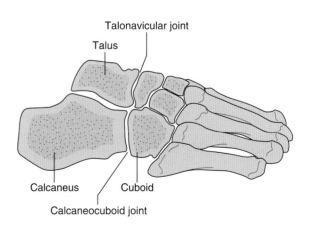

Figure 13.2 Midtarsal joint.

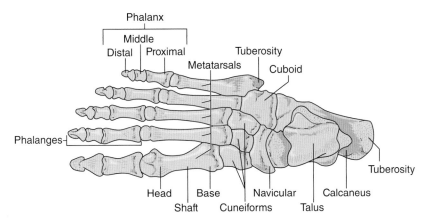

Figure 13.3 Anterior view of the foot.

Metatarsophalangeal Joints

The phalanges and metatarsals together form the forefoot. The metatarsophalangeal (MTP) joint is a diarthrodial condyloid joint. Each MTP consists of the convex head of the metatarsal and concave base of the proximal phalanx. Each MTP is supported by 2 collateral ligaments: medial and lateral. The fibrous joint capsules surround the joints and are attached to the margins of the articular surfaces. Dorsally, they are thin and may be separated from the tendons of the long extensors by small bursae. The capsule is inseparable from the deep surfaces of the plantar and collateral ligaments. The plantar aponeurosis blends with the metatarsal heads for further plantar reinforcement.

Interphalangeal Joints

The interphalangeal joints are diarthrodial hinge joints. The joint consists of the convex head of the proximal phalanx and the concave base of the distal phalanx. The articular capsule surrounds the entire joint and is reinforced by a medial and lateral collateral ligament. The plantar surface of the articular capsule is strengthened to form a fibrous plate, called the plantar ligament. Dorsally,

the extensor tendon that attaches on the distal phalanx helps to reinforce the joint.

Joint Kinematics

The joints of the foot are numerous, and joint motion traverses multiple planes. Hyper- or hypo-mobility of a single joint influences joint mobility elsewhere. The clinician must have a good understanding of the intricacies of these joints in order to treat this area effectively.

Subtalar Joint

The subtalar joint is a uniaxial joint that produces motion—supination and pronation—in 3 planes. The axis of rotation can vary among individuals but averages around 42° above the AP axis from the horizontal plane and 23° medial to the AP axis from the sagittal plane (figure 13.4). One way to identify this clinically is that the axis is perpendicular to a line that bisects the sinus tarsi and the sustentaculum tali. Open chain triplane pronation consists of calcaneal eversion (frontal plane), abduction (transverse plane), and dorsiflexion (sagittal plane). Triplane supination consists

---

Clinical Tips

The articulation between the cuneiforms and the metatarsals, clinically, is referred to as the Lisfranc joint. This can be the site for a fracture/dislocation called a Lisfranc fracture, ligamentous trauma, or Lisfranc sprain. These injuries can cause extreme pain and long-term issues if not treated appropriately.

Clinical Tips

Turf toe is an injury to the soft tissue structures about the MTP joint. Most commonly it is a sprain to the collateral ligaments that support this joint. The mechanism of injury is a forcible hyperextension of the great toe, such as when pushing off into a sprint and having the toe get stuck flat on the ground.

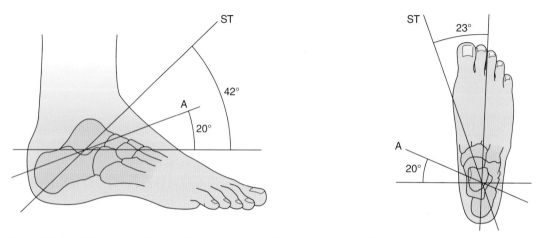

Figure 13.4   Orientation of axes of rotation of the subtalar joint. A = ankle joint axis; ST = subtalar joint axis.

of calcaneal inversion (frontal plane), adduction (transverse plane), plantarflexion (sagittal plane). In weight bearing, this triplane motion is described as the talus moving on the calcaneus. Pronation is described as talar plantarflexion, adduction, and calcaneal eversion. Supination is described as talar dorsiflexion, abduction, and calcaneal inversion (figure 13.5).

Midtarsal Joint

There are 2 joint axes described for the midtarsal joint. One is longitudinal and runs 15° upward from the transverse plane and 9° medially from longitudinal reference. Inversion and eversion occur about the longitudinal axis. The second axis is oblique and runs 52° upward from the transverse plane and 57° medially from the frontal plane. Flexion and extension occur about the oblique axis. The calcaneocuboid and talonavicular joints allow for slight gliding motion in 3 planes and follow closely the motion of the subtalar joint.

When the midtarsal axes are parallel, as with foot pronation, the entire foot becomes mobile or flexible (figure 13.6). When the axes are nonparallel, as with foot supination, the entire foot becomes rigid.

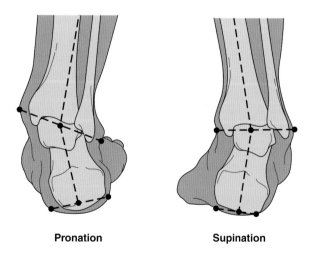

Pronation   **Supination**

Figure 13.5   Motions of the subtalar joint.

The foot is an amazing complex. It has the ability to be flexible for absorbing ground reaction forces. This occurs early in the gait cycle, specifically during loading response up until the beginning of midstance. It then becomes a rigid lever for push-off during the latter part of midstance until the foot leaves the ground.

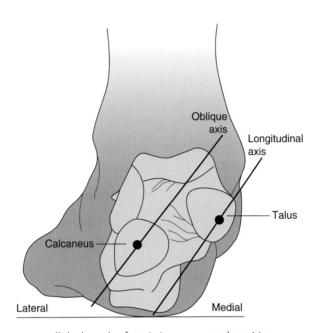

Figure 13.6 Midtarsal axes are parallel when the foot is in a pronated position.

Tarsometatarsal Joints

Along with the midtarsal joint, the tarsometatarsals are responsible for counteracting the motion of the rearfoot during pronation and supination. This counteraction helps to keep the foot on the ground.

Metatarsophalangeal Joints

The MTP joints are biaxial with 2 degrees of freedom: flexion/extension and abduction/adduction. Flexion and extension occurs about a medial/longitudinal axis in the sagittal plane. Abduction and adduction occur about a vertical axis in the horizontal plane. Open chain motion follows the convex-concave rule; MTP extension involves a dorsal glide of the concave phalanx on the convex metatarsal, and MTP flexion requires a plantar glide of the phalanx. MTP abduction/adduction consists of the phalanx gliding in the same direction as bone movement. During closed chain motion, the phalanx is pinned to the ground and the convex metatarsal will move opposite bone movement. For example, great toe extension involves the metatarsal gliding plantarly on the fixed proximal phalanx.

Interphalangeal Joints

The interphalangeal joints have 1 degree of freedom about a medial/lateral axis. The movement at this joint is flexion and extension. Arthrokinematic motion of flexion and extension is the same as the MTP.

FOOT JOINT ARTHROLOGY

Articular surfaces	Closed packed position	Resting position	Capsular pattern	ROM norms	End-feel
Subtalar joint					
3 facets on inferior talus with 3 facets on superior calcaneus	Supination	Midway between supination and pronation	Inversion limited more than pronation	Calcaneal inversion: 30° Calcaneal eversion: 15°	Tissue stretch in both directions; eversion can be hard if calcaneus hits sinus tarsi
Midtarsal joints					
Calcaneocuboid: sellar articulation between calcaneus and cuboid Talonavicular: convex head of talus and concave navicular	Supination	Midway between supination and pronation	Both joints: limitation of dorsiflexion > plantar flexion > adduction and internal rotation	Not defined	Tissue stretch in both directions
Tarsometatarsal joints					
Concave base of metatarsals and cuneiforms or cuboid	Pronation	Midway between supination and pronation	Equal limitation in all directions	Not defined	Tissue stretch in all directions
Metatarsophalangeal joints					
Convex distal metatarsal and the concave proximal phalanx	Full extension	Midway between flexion and extension	Greater limitation in extension than flexion	Flexion: 20° Extension: 70° Abduction: 10°	Tissue stretch in all directions
Interphalangeal joints					
Convex proximal phalanx and the concave distal phalanx	Full extension	Out of full extension	Flexion more limited than extension	PIP flexion: 90° DIP flexion: 40° Great toe extension: 70°	Tissue stretch in all directions

Distraction

VIDEO 13.1 **in the web study guide shows this technique.**

Client position: Prone with foot off treatment table, subtalar joint in resting position.

Clinician position: Sitting at foot of treatment table facing the plantar surface of client's foot.

Stabilization: Inferior stabilizing hand grips the talus at the dorsal surface of lower leg with the hand's web space.

Mobilization: Superior manipulating hand grips the calcaneus on the posterior surface of lower leg with hand's ulnar border and moves the calcaneus distally.

Goal of technique: To increase general ankle motion.

Note: This technique can also be performed with the client supine.

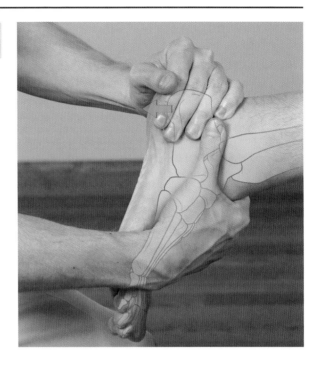

Lateral Glide

Client position: For the right limb, right side-lying with leg supported on treatment table with towel or pillow.

Clinician position: Standing at end of treatment table facing side of client in a walk-stance position.

Stabilization: The clinician stabilizes the talus with the web space of the left hand and places base of the right hand on the side of the calcaneus medially while wrapping fingers around the plantar surface of client's right foot.

Mobilization: Clinician applies a lateral glide. Initial pressure should be applied gently; increase amplitude and depth of the movement if no pain response occurs.

Goal of technique: To improve lateral glide, which will improve eversion.

Note: This technique can also be performed with the client supine or prone.

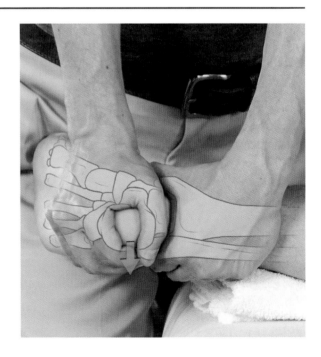

Medial Glide

Client position: For the right limb, left side-lying with right leg supported on treatment table with towel or pillow.

Clinician position: Standing at end of treatment table facing side of client in a walk-stance position.

Stabilization: The clinician stabilizes the talus with the web space of the right hand and places base of left hand on side of the calcaneus laterally while wrapping fingers around the plantar surface of client's right foot.

Mobilization: Clinician applies a medial glide. Initial pressure should be applied gently; increase amplitude and depth of the movement if no pain response occurs.

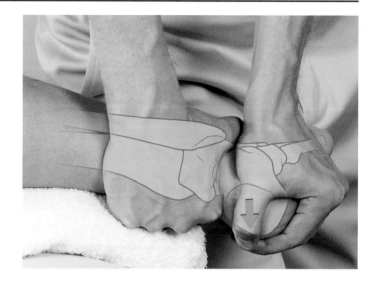

Goal of technique: To improve medial glide, which will improve inversion.

Note: This technique can also be performed with the client supine or prone.

Calcaneal Rocking

 VIDEO 13.2 in the web study guide shows this technique.

Client position: Side-lying with mobilizing foot on top.

Clinician position: Sitting on treatment table with back to client.

Stabilization: The client's knee is flexed; the posterior thigh is stabilized by the clinician's trunk.

Mobilization: Clinician grasps client's calcaneus with thumbs forming a V over the lateral aspect of client's calcaneus. Clinician's forearms are in the direction of the applied force. Distraction can be performed in isolation or with a medial and lateral glide.

Goal of technique: To aid in the motion of pronation and supination.

Note: The client can be supine with the clinician sitting in front of the client.

Navicular Dorsal (Anterior) Glide

Client position: Prone with knee flexed to 90° with foot in resting position.

Clinician position: Facing the lateral aspect of client's affected foot.

Stabilization: The stabilizing hand grasps neck of the talus at the dorsal surface of foot with hand's web space.

Mobilization: The manipulating hand's thumb is placed on the plantar surface of the navicular, while index finger is on its dorsal surface. The navicular is glided dorsally.

Goal of technique: To assist with midtarsal inversion (along the longitudinal axis) and midtarsal dorsiflexion (along the oblique axis).

Note: A variety of hand positions can be used to accomplish the same mobilization technique.

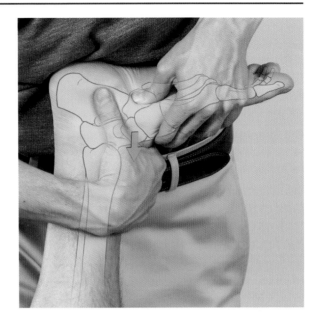

Navicular Dorsolateral Glide

Client position: Prone with knee flexed to 90° with foot in resting position.

Clinician position: Facing the lateral aspect of client's affected foot.

Stabilization: The stabilizing hand grasps neck of the talus at the dorsal surface of foot with hand's web space.

Mobilization: The mobilizing hand is positioned with web space over the plantar surface of the navicular. It glides the medial navicular in a dorsolateral direction, rotating the navicular into a more supinated position.

Goal of technique: To assist with midtarsal inversion (along the longitudinal axis) and midtarsal dorsiflexion (along the oblique axis).

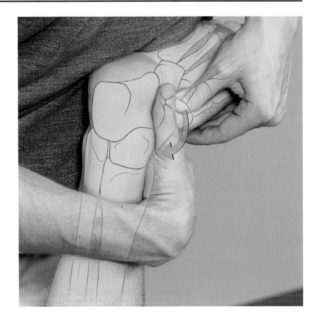

Navicular Plantar (Posterior) Glide

VIDEO 13.3 in the web study guide shows this technique.

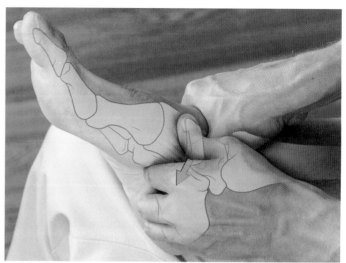

Client position: Supine with ankle and foot joint in resting position supported by the clinician's thigh.

Clinician position: Seated on treatment table facing the medial aspect of foot to be treated.

Stabilization: The stabilizing hand grasps neck of the talus at the dorsal surface of foot with web space and fingers. Foot may be placed against clinician's trunk for additional stabilization.

Mobilization: The manipulating hand is positioned on the navicular with thumb on the dorsal surface and index finger on the plantar surface. Hand glides the navicular in a plantar direction.

Goal of technique: To increase midtarsal eversion along the longitudinal axis and midtarsal plantarflexion.

Navicular Plantarmedial Glide

Client position: Supine with ankle and foot joint in resting position supported by the clinician's thigh.

Clinician position: Seated on treatment table facing the lateral aspect of foot to be treated.

Stabilization: The stabilizing hand grasps neck of the talus at the dorsal surface of foot with web space and fingers. Foot may be placed against the clinician's trunk for additional stabilization.

Mobilization: The manipulating hand is positioned with web space over dorsal surface of the navicular. It glides the medial navicular in a plantarmedial direction, rotating the navicular into a more pronated position.

Goal of technique: To increase midtarsal eversion along the longitudinal axis and midtarsal plantarflexion.

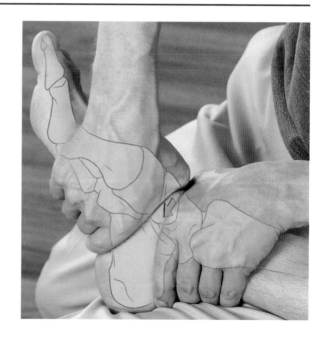

Cuboid Dorsal (Anterior) Glide

Client position: Prone with knee flexed to 90° with foot in resting position.

Clinician position: Standing and facing the medial aspect of client's affected foot.

Stabilization: The stabilizing hand grips the calcaneus on the posterior aspect with web space and fingers.

Mobilization: The manipulating hand is placed on the cuboid with thumb on plantar surface and index finger on dorsal surface. It glides the cuboid in a dorsal direction.

Goal of technique: To assist with midtarsal eversion (along the longitudinal axis) and midtarsal dorsiflexion (along the oblique axis).

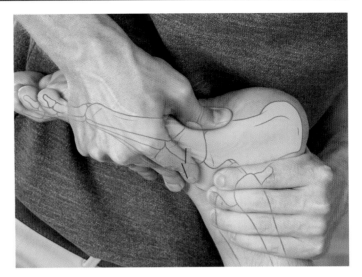

Cuboid Dorsolateral Glide

Client position: Prone with knee flexed to 90° with foot in resting position.

Clinician position: Standing and facing the medial aspect of client's affected foot.

Stabilization: The stabilizing hand grips the calcaneus on the plantar aspect with web space and wraps index and ring finger around the surface of the cuboid.

Mobilization: The manipulating hand is placed with web space on the cuboid's plantar surface. Hand glides the cuboid in a dorsolateral direction, rotating the cuboid into a more pronated position.

Goal of technique: To assist with midtarsal eversion (along the longitudinal axis) and midtarsal dorsiflexion (along the oblique axis).

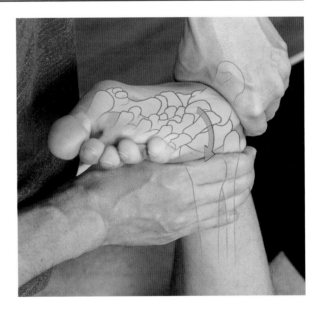

Cuboid Plantar (Posterior) Glide

Client position: Supine with the joint in its resting position supported by the clinician's thigh.

Clinician position: Standing and facing the medial aspect of client's affected foot.

Stabilization: The stabilizing hand grips the distal ankle joint. Foot may be placed against clinician's trunk for additional stabilization.

Mobilization: The manipulating hand is placed with thumb on dorsal surface of cuboid and index finger on plantar surface of cuboid. Hand mobilizes cuboid in a plantar direction.

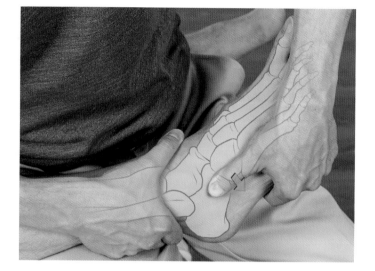

Goal of technique: To increase midtarsal inversion along the longitudinal axis and midtarsal plantarflexion along the oblique axis.

Cuboid Plantarmedial Glide

Client position: Supine with the joint in its resting position supported by the clinician's thigh.

Clinician position: Sitting and facing the medial aspect of client's affected foot.

Stabilization: The stabilizing hand grips the calcaneus on the plantar surface of foot. The foot may be placed against clinician's trunk for additional stabilization.

Mobilization: The manipulating hand is placed with web space over dorsal surface of cuboid. Hand mobilizes cuboid in a plantarmedial direction, rotating cuboid into a more supinated position.

Goal of technique: To increase midtarsal inversion along the longitudinal axis and midtarsal plantarflexion along the oblique axis.

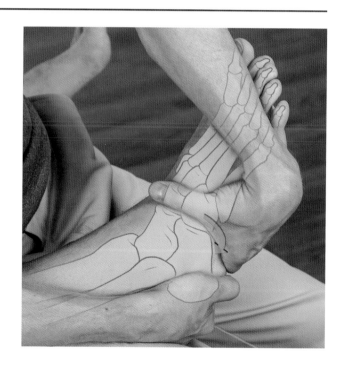

Cuboid Manipulation

VIDEO 13.4 **in the web study guide shows this technique.**

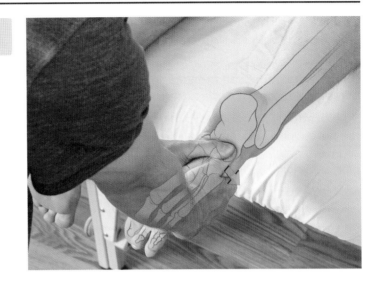

Client position: Prone near edge of treatment table with knee bent to 70°.

Clinician position: Standing facing the plantar surface of the foot.

Stabilization: Clinician places fingers in an interlocking position over the dorsum of client's foot. Clinician's thumbs are placed on the plantar surface of the cuboid.

Mobilization: The client's ankle is dorsiflexed to approximately 0°. The manipulation is performed by extending knee, plantar flexing ankle, with slight supination of the subtalar joint. Clinician's thumbs apply a thrust force to the cuboid with stabilization of foot by interlocked fingers.

Goal of technique: To improve mobility of the calcaneocuboid joint or relocate a plantarflexed cuboid.

Note: This technique can also be used on the talonavicular joint.

Dorsal (Anterior) Glide

Client position: Supine with the joint in its resting position supported by the clinician's thigh.

Clinician position: Sitting and facing the dorsal aspect of foot to be treated.

Stabilization: The stabilizing hand grasps the tarsal bone with thumb on the dorsal surface of foot and index finger on the plantar surface of foot.

Mobilization: The manipulating hand grips the metatarsal with thumb on the dorsal surface of foot and index finger on plantar surface of foot. Hand glides the first metatarsal in a dorsal direction on the first cuneiform, the second metatarsal in a dorsal direction on the second cuneiform, the third metatarsal in a dorsal direction on the cuboid, and the fourth and fifth metatarsals in a dorsal direction on the cuboid.

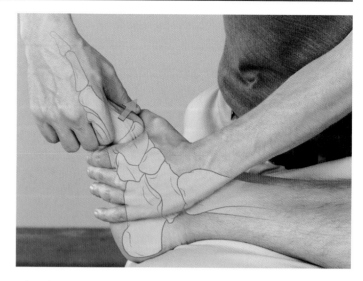

Goal of technique: To increase dorsiflexion.

Note: There is very minimal movement in these joints.

Plantar (Posterior) Glide

Client position: Supine with the joint in its resting position supported by the clinician's thigh.

Clinician position: Sitting and facing the dorsal aspect of foot to be treated.

Stabilization: The stabilizing hand grasps the tarsal bone with thumb on the dorsal surface of foot and index finger on the plantar surface of metatarsal.

Mobilization: The manipulating hand grips the metatarsal with thumb on the dorsal surface of foot and index finger on the plantar surface of phalanx. Hand glides the first metatarsal in a plantar direction on the first cuneiform, the second metatarsal in a plantar direction on the second cuneiform, the third metatarsal in a plantar direction on the cuboid, and the fourth and fifth metatarsals in a plantar direction on the cuboid.

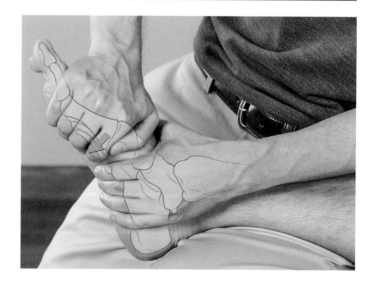

Goal of technique: To increase plantarflexion.

Note: There is very minimal movement in these joints.

Distraction

Client position: Supine with the joint in its resting position supported by the clinician's thigh.

Clinician position: Sitting and facing the dorsal aspect of foot to be treated.

Stabilization: The stabilizing hand grasps the tarsal bone with thumb on dorsal surface of foot and index finger on plantar surface of foot.

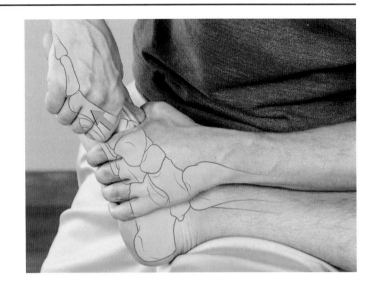

Mobilization: The manipulating hand grips the metatarsal with the thumb on the dorsal surface of the foot and the index finger on the plantar surface of the foot. The clinician applies a distraction force.

Goal of technique: To improve mobility of the tarsometatarsal joint.

Notes: A wedge may be used to stabilize the foot. This technique can be used on any of the tarsometatarsal joints.

Distraction

VIDEO 13.5 in the web study guide shows this technique.

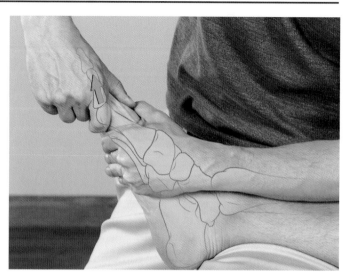

Client position: Supine with the joint in its resting position supported by the clinician's thigh.

Clinician position: Sitting and facing the dorsal aspect of foot to be treated.

Stabilization: The stabilizing hand grasps head of metatarsal with thumb on dorsal aspect and index finger on plantar surface of foot.

Mobilization: The manipulating hand grasps the proximal end of the proximal phalanx to be manipulated with thumb on dorsal surface and index finger on plantar surface of foot. Hand moves base of the proximal phalanx distally.

Goal of technique: To improve general mobility of the joint or relieve pain.

Note: A surgical glove or dysum can be used to obtain increased grip on the phalanx.

Dorsal (Anterior) Glide

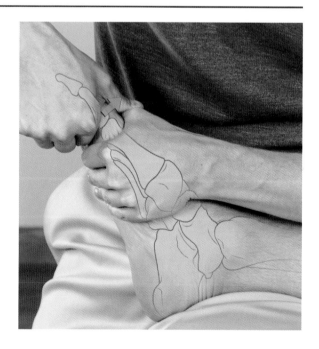

Client position: Supine with the joint in its resting position supported by the clinician's thigh.

Clinician position: Sitting and facing the dorsal aspect of foot to be treated.

Stabilization: The stabilizing hand grasps head of metatarsal with thumb on dorsal aspect and index finger on plantar surface of metatarsal.

Mobilization: The manipulating hand grasps proximal end of proximal phalanx to be manipulated with thumb on dorsal surface and index finger on plantar surface of phalanx. Hand moves base of the proximal phalanx dorsally.

Goal of technique: To improve toe extension.

Note: A surgical glove or dysum can be used to obtain increased grip on the phalanx.

Plantar (Posterior) Glide

Client position: Supine with the joint in its resting position supported by the clinician's thigh.

Clinician position: Sitting and facing the dorsal aspect of foot to be treated.

Stabilization: The stabilizing hand grasps head of metatarsal with thumb on dorsal aspect and index finger on plantar surface of metatarsal.

Mobilization: The manipulating hand grasps proximal end of proximal phalanx to be manipulated with thumb on dorsal surface and index finger on plantar surface of phalanx. Hand moves base of the proximal phalanx plantarly.

Goal of technique: To improve toe flexion.

Note: A surgical glove or dysum can be used to obtain increased grip on the phalanx.

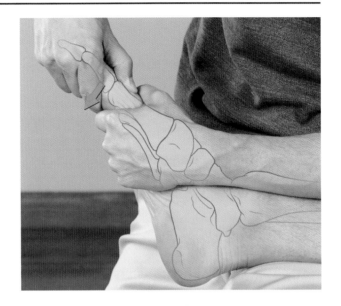

Medial Glide

VIDEO 13.6 **in the web study guide shows this technique.**

Client position: Supine with the joint in its resting position supported by the clinician's thigh.

Clinician position: Sitting and facing the dorsal aspect of foot to be treated.

Stabilization: The stabilizing hand grasps head of metatarsal with thumb on lateral aspect and index finger on medial surface of metatarsal.

Mobilization: The manipulating hand grasps the proximal phalanx to be manipulated on the medial and lateral surfaces and glides it in a medial direction.

Goal of technique: To improve medial glide of the joint.

Note: A surgical glove or dysum can be used to obtain increased grip on the phalanx.

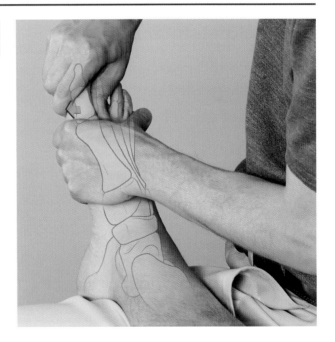

Lateral Glide

Client position: Supine with the joint in its resting position supported by the clinician's thigh.

Clinician position: Sitting and facing the dorsal aspect of foot to be treated.

Stabilization: The stabilizing hand grasps head of metatarsal with thumb on lateral aspect and index finger on medial surface of metatarsal.

Mobilization: The manipulating hand grasps the proximal phalanx to be manipulated on the medial and lateral surfaces and glides it in a lateral direction.

Goal of technique: To improve lateral glide of the joint.

Note: A surgical glove or dysum can be used to obtain increased grip on the phalanx.

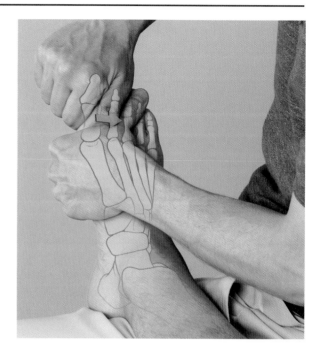

Sesamoid Mobilization

Client position: Supine with foot relaxed.

Clinician position: Standing or sitting and facing client's foot. The clinician places a thumb on the proximal aspect of the sesamoid.

Stabilization: The clinician's cranial hand grasps the distal first metatarsal with a firm grip.

Mobilization: The clinician applies a distal glide that causes the sesamoid to reach the end range of available motion.

Goal of technique: To improve joint mobility in individuals with hallux limitus.

Note: Care must be taken not to compress the sesamoid against the head of the first metatarsal.

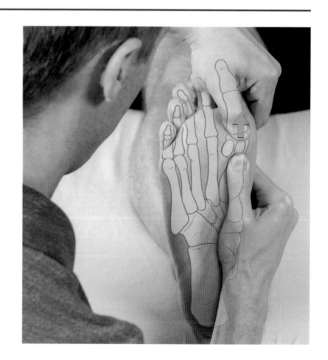

Intermetatarsal Mobilization

VIDEO 13.7 **in the web study guide shows this technique.**

Client position: Supine with the joint in its resting position.

Clinician position: Sitting and facing the plantar aspect of foot to be treated.

Stabilization: The resting leg of client helps stabilize the limb.

Mobilization: Clinician's hands grasp forefoot so fingers are on the dorsal aspect and thumbs are on the plantar aspect of foot. Thumbs push dorsally against fingers serving as a fulcrum to create a bending motion of forefoot. Work each of the intermetatarsal joints.

Goal of technique: To improve mobility of the forefoot.

Note: The motion can be performed in a plantar direction using the fingers as the mobilizing force and the thumbs as the fulcrum.

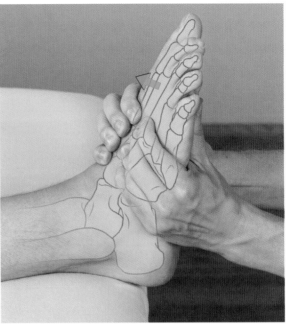

Distraction

Client position: Supine with the joint in resting position supported by the clinician's thigh.

Clinician position: Sitting and facing the dorsal aspect of foot to be treated.

Stabilization: The stabilizing hand grips distal end of proximal phalanx of joint to be treated with thumb on dorsal surface and index finger on plantar surface of foot.

Mobilization: The manipulating hand grips proximal end of the distal phalanx of joint to be treated with thumb on dorsal surface and index finger on plantar surface of foot. Hand distracts the distal phalanx distally.

Goal of technique: To improve general mobility of the joint or relieve pain.

Note: This technique may be helpful for stiff toe mobility.

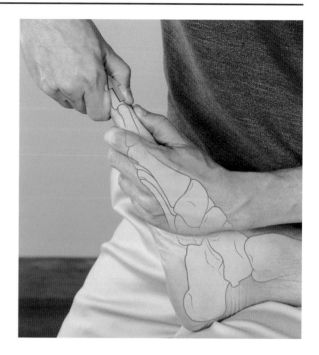

Dorsal (Anterior) Glide

Client position: Supine with the joint in resting position supported by the clinician's thigh.

Clinician position: Sitting and facing the dorsal aspect of foot to be treated.

Stabilization: The stabilizing hand grips distal end of proximal phalanx of joint to be treated with thumb on dorsal surface and index finger on plantar surface of foot.

Mobilization: The manipulating hand grips the proximal end of the distal phalanx of joint to be treated with thumb on dorsal surface and index finger on plantar surface of foot. Hand mobilizes the distal phalanx dorsally.

Goal of technique: To improve toe extension.

Note: This technique may be helpful for stiff toe mobility.

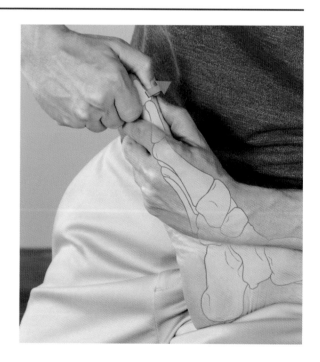

Plantar (Posterior) Glide

Client position: Supine with the joint in resting position supported by the clinician's thigh.

Clinician position: Sitting and facing the dorsal aspect of foot to be treated.

Stabilization: The stabilizing hand grips distal end of proximal phalanx of joint to be treated with thumb on dorsal surface and index finger on plantar surface of foot.

Mobilization: The manipulating hand grips proximal end of distal phalanx of joint to be treated with thumb on dorsal surface and index finger on plantar surface of foot. Hand mobilizes the distal phalanx plantarly.

Goal of technique: To improve toe extension.

Note: This technique may be helpful for stiff toe mobility.

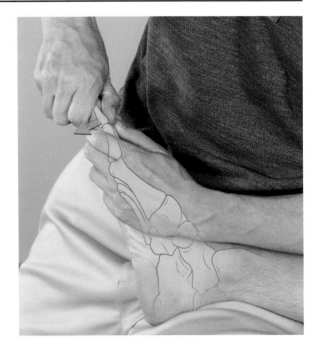

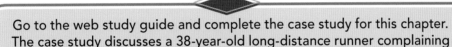

Go to the web study guide and complete the case study for this chapter. The case study discusses a 38-year-old long-distance runner complaining of plantar heel pain.

EVIDENCE FOR MANUAL THERAPY OF VARIOUS FOOT PATHOLOGIES

Study	Clients	Intervention and comparison (if any)	Outcome(s)
Utilization of thrust and nonthrust mobilization for plantar fasciopathy: Grade C
Celik et al., 2016 (Level 2b)	43 clients with plantar fasciitis	Clients randomly assigned to either joint mobilization and stretching or steroid injections.	FAAM, VAS were evaluated at baseline, 3, 6, 12 weeks, and 1 year. At 12 weeks and 1 year, joint mob group significantly improved over steroid group.
Cleland et al., 2009 (Level 1b)	60 clients with primary complaint of plantar heel pain	Clients randomly assigned to 1 of 2 groups; group 1 received electrotherapy and stretching; group 2 received soft tissue mobilization and joint mobilization to subtalar joint.	Manual therapy group improved at 4 weeks, maintained improvement up to 6 months using the following outcome measures: FAAM, LEFS, GRoC.
Shasua et al., 2015 (Level 1b)	46 clients with plantar fasciitis aged 23 to 73 years	Clients randomly assigned to intervention or control group. Both groups received 8 treatments of stretching and US; intervention group also received mobilization of ankle and midfoot.	No significant difference in NPRS, LEFS, algometry, and df ROM was found between groups although both groups improved in all measures.
Utilization of thrust and nonthrust mobilization for cuboid syndrome: Grade D
Jennings & Davies, 2005 (Level 4)	7 clients following a lateral ankle sprain with chief complaint of lateral ankle/midfoot pain	Cuboid manipulation was applied to each client.	All 7 clients returned to sports activities following 1 to 2 treatments.
Utilization of thrust and nonthrust mobilization for metatarsalgia: Grade B
Govender et al., 2007 (Level 1c)	40 clients with Morton's neuroma Average age = 51 years	Mobilization and manipulation for foot and ankle vs. placebo (detuned ultrasound); 6 treatments over 3 weeks.	Significantly in favor for manual therapy: NPRS and algometry vs. placebo.
Petersen et al., 2003 (Level 2b)	40 clients with metatarsalgia Average age = 49.5 years	Manual therapy of foot and ankle (mob, HVLA: especially intermetatarsal glide, first MTPJ, etc.) vs. placebo (detuned ultrasound); 8 treatments over 4 weeks.	Significantly in favor for manual therapy vs. placebo for: SFMPQ, NPRS, FFI, and algometry. Note: placebo clients started with higher level of pain.

Study	Clients	Intervention and comparison (if any)	Outcome(s)
Utilization of thrust and nonthrust mobilization for hallux rigidus: Grade B			
Shamus et al., 2004 (Level 1c)	20 clients with first MPJ pain and loss of ROM	Clients randomly divided into 2 groups. Both groups received whirlpool, ultrasound, first MPJ mobilizations, calf/hamstring stretching, marble pick-up exercise, cold packs, and electrical stimulation. The intervention group received sesamoid mobilizations, flexor hallucis strengthening exercises, and gait training.	Following 12 therapy sessions, the experimental group achieved significantly greater MPJ extension ROM and flexor hallucis strength and had significantly lower pain levels as compared to the control group.
Utilization of thrust and nonthrust mobilization for hallux abducto valgus: Grade B			
Brantingham et al., 2005 (Level 1c)	60 clients with HAV Average age = 50.1 years	Clients randomly assigned to 1 of 2 groups. Group 1 received mobilization and manipulation to the hallux and foot. Group 2 received nontherapeutic action potential therapy. 6 treatments over 3 weeks.	Significantly in favor for manual therapy for ↓NPRS, ↓disability, ↑function with FFI compared to placebo group.

FAAM = foot and ankle measure; LEFS = lower extremity functional scale; GRoC = global rate of change; VAS = visual analog scale; US = ultrasound; NPRS = numeric pain rating scale; df = dorsiflexion; ROM = range of motion; MPJ = metatarsophalangeal joint; HVLA = high-velocity, low-amplitude thrust; MTPJ = metatarsophalangeal joint; SFMPQ = short form McGill pain questionnaire; HAV = hallux abducto valgus; FFI = foot function index

APPENDIX

Self-Mobilizations

General Instructions for Integration of Self-Mobilization Techniques Into a Home Program

- The clinician should be confident in client's ability to safely and independently perform the self-mobilizations.
- Clients should independently demonstrate the technique(s) properly before they are prescribed.
- It is ideal to have some form of warm-up (e.g., 5–8 minutes of walking or riding a bicycle for lower extremity joints) prior to self-mobilizations.
- Static stretching of surrounding muscles for a few sets of 30 to 60 seconds may provide benefit.
- Clients should complete the prescribed self-mobilizations using repetitions, loads, and durations prescribed by the clinician.
- Exercises into newly gained ranges of motion may provide benefit. For example, clients can perform end-range isometric or full-arc isotonic exercises as prescribed by clinician(s).

Clinical Tip

Muscle activity around joints attempting to be mobilized will typically overpower the force of self-nonthrusts. To optimize the effectiveness of self-nonthrusts, clients should attempt to relax the muscles around the joints being mobilized. For example, in the hip, shifting the weight of the body onto the side not being mobilized might help muscles around the target hip relax and the joint to distract or glide as desired.

Mouth Opening (Bilateral TMJ Protrusion)

Client position: Seated, preferably with back against a stable surface.

Stabilization: Client's body serves as stabilization.

Mobilization: Client grasps chin between thumb and index finger and glides the mandible down, as tolerated.

Goal of technique: To improve mouth opening.

Note: This technique can be biased toward one side for a lateral excursion technique similar to the following technique.

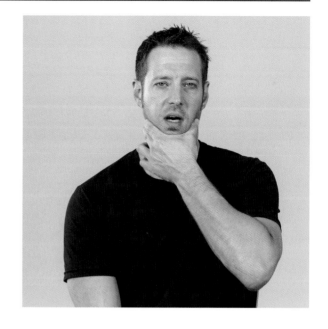

Mandible Lateral Excursion (Lateral Jaw Movement)

Client position: Seated.

Stabilization: Client's body serves as stabilization.

Mobilization: Client uses heel of hand to glide mandible contralaterally, as tolerated.

Goal of technique: To promote protrusion on the side being treated.

Note: Client may also use the other hand and grasp the mandible with the fingers to provide the same force.

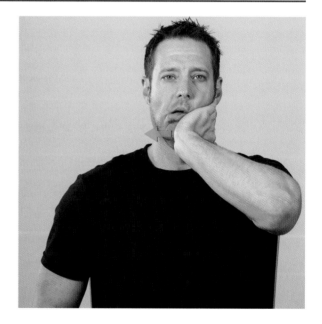

C2-C7 Rotation (Opening Contralateral Facet)

Client position: Seated with second and third fingers of hand opposite the side to be mobilized purchasing the target facet joint on contralateral side of cervical rotation. For increased comfort and stabilization, client may lean back against a solid surface.

Stabilization: Client's body serves as stabilization.

Mobilization: Guide motion along the plane of the facet joint with fingers purchased on the facet joint. The direction of mobilization is toward the ipsilateral eye.

Goal of technique: To supplement treatment techniques aimed at improving cervical rotation.

Note: The cervical spine can be in neutral or degrees of flexion. Increasing flexion will facilitate up and forward motion of the target facet joint.

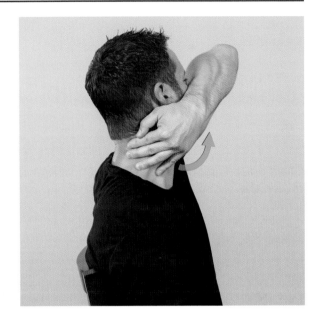

C2-C7 Rotation (Closing Ipsilateral Facet)

Client position: Seated with second and third fingers of hand opposite side to be mobilized stabilizing the target facet joint on ipsilateral side of cervical rotation. For increased comfort and stabilization, client may lean back against a solid surface.

Stabilization: Client's second and third fingers purchasing the facet joint serve as stabilization.

Mobilization: Rotate head in direction of restriction, maintaining stabilization.

Goal of technique: To supplement treatment techniques aimed at improving cervical rotation.

Note: The cervical spine can be in neutral or degrees of extension. Increasing extension will facilitate down and back movement of the ipsilateral facet joint targeted.

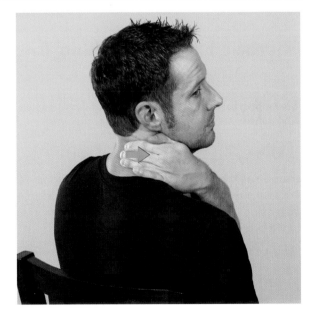

First Rib Inferior Glide

VIDEO A.1 **in the web study guide shows this technique.**

Client position: Seated.

Stabilization: Client's body serves as stabilization.

Mobilization: A towel or bed sheet is tucked into armpit on the ipsilateral side and placed over shoulder as close to cervical spine as possible. Client grasps sheet with both hands and angles it toward the contralateral hip. Client takes a deep breath, pulling sheet down toward the contralateral hip. Client continues to pull sheet toward hip while exhaling. This cycle is repeated as tolerated.

Goal of technique: To assist with pain-free breathing and mobilization of the first rib.

Note: If the sheet is long enough, client can place the end under the ipsilateral buttock versus the armpit. This will allow client to relax the ipsilateral arm and provide increased mechanical advantage for the mobilization.

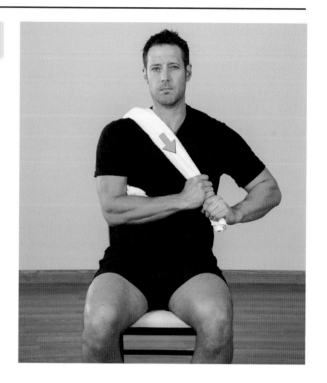

Thoracic Extension With a Towel

Client position: Seated in a chair.

Stabilization: Client rolls a sheet lengthwise, places a towel through the sheet at the midpoint to make a Y, sits on the ends of the sheet, and holds the ends of the towel in front of the body.

Mobilization: The junction of the sheet and towel is placed over the segment to be mobilized into extension. Client performs a cervical retraction while pulling the ends of the towel forward.

Goal of technique: To improve thoracic extension at the target segment.

Note: This technique works best for upper- or mid-thoracic segments.

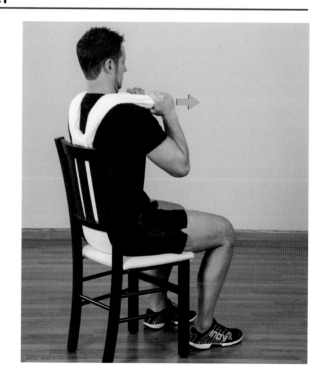

Mid-Thoracic Extension With a Chair

Client position: Seated in a chair with hands behind head and hypomobile region of the thoracic spine against the back of a chair or table.

Stabilization: The chair or table provides the needed stabilization.

Mobilization: Client leans back against the top of the chair or edge of the table to fulcrum at the desired level of mobilization.

Goal of technique: To improve thoracic extension at the target segment.

Note: Client might need to sit forward or back in the chair to fulcrum at the desired segment.

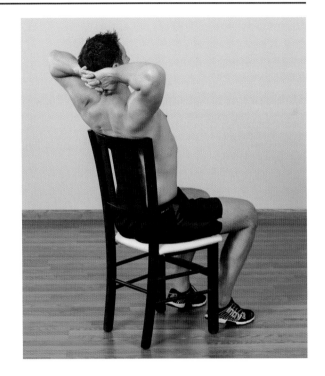

Thoracic Foam Rolling

Client position: Lying on a foam roller placed perpendicular to spine, with knees and hips slightly flexed and feet on floor.

Stabilization: Client's feet placed shoulder-width apart provide stability.

Mobilization: Client rolls up and down the length of the thoracic spine as tolerated, targeting hypomobile segments as needed.

Goal of technique: To improve general mobility of the thoracic spine.

Note: Client should maintain a neutral spine position throughout the technique.

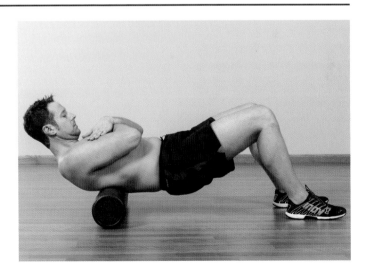

Lumbar Extension

Client position: Standing or seated with one thumb over another on the inferior spinous process of the hypomobile segment.

Stabilization: Client provides an anteriorly directed pressure with thumbs over the spinous process for stabilization.

Mobilization: Client actively extends spine to end range, maintaining stabilization.

Goal of technique: To improve segmental lumbar extension.

Notes: To direct mobilization to a single facet joint, ipsilateral rotation and/or rotation with extension can be performed with this technique. If mobilization of a single facet joint is desired, the thumb-over-thumb stabilization pressure can also be applied directly to that facet joint.

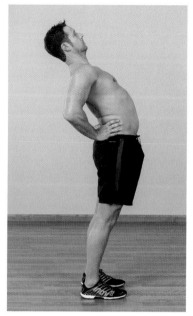
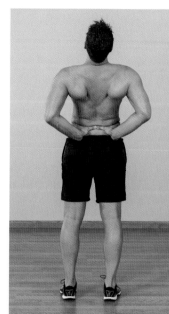

Glenohumeral Posterior Glide

Client position: Standing with the uninvolved side's hand over the anterior portion of the target glenohumeral joint.

Stabilization: Client's shoulder connected to the axial spine provides its own stabilization.

Mobilization: Client actively abducts shoulder while applying an anterior-to-posterior force to the humeral head.

Goal of technique: To improve posterior glide of the moving humeral head.

Note: This technique is done with active shoulder abduction to directly assist client's functional movement.

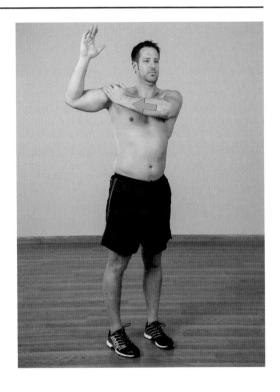

Wrist and Hand Distraction

Client position: Seated with forearm in neutral rotation and resting on a table, with hand just off table.

Stabilization: The forearm is stabilized by the table.

Mobilization: Grip proximal row of wrist and pull this row of carpal bones away from stabilized forearm.

Goals of technique: To improve general mobility at this joint. Also, oscillation of the distraction might decrease pain.

Note: Instruct client to gradually increase the distraction force to this joint complex.

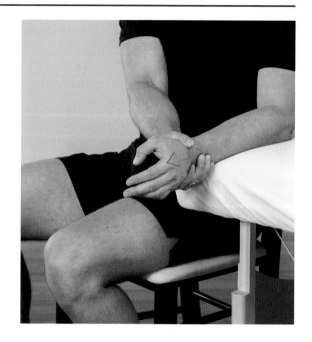

Anterior Glide at the Radiocarpal Joint

Client position: Standing with mobilizing hand flat on table and elbow straight.

Stabilization: Keeping the palm against the table provides sufficient stabilization.

Mobilization: The top hand covers the bottom hand as close to the radiocarpal joint as possible. Apply pressure through the upright forearm in a downward and posterior direction. At the same time, client can work to increase wrist extension by moving forearm toward fingers.

Goal of technique: To increase wrist extension.

Note: Approximately 70° of wrist extension is normal.

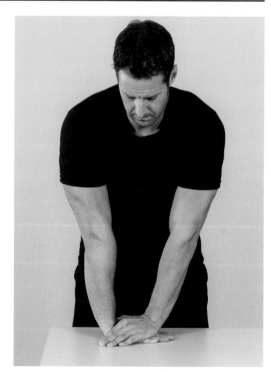

MCP or Phalangeal Distractions

Client position: Seated with forearm and hand in neutral rotation and resting on a table.

Stabilization: Keeping force against the table with the mobilizing side forearm aids stabilization of the hand.

Mobilization: Grasp the distal segment of the joint to be manipulated with the other hand. Gently pull the segment in a linear direction away from the proximal segment, creating a distraction of the joint.

Goals of technique: To improve general joint mobility. Also, oscillation of the distraction might decrease pain.

Note: A manipulative thrust may be applied in a similar manner.

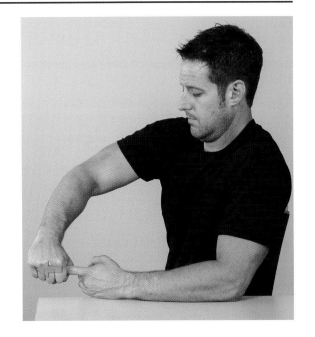

MCP or Phalangeal Glide

Client position: Seated with forearm and hand in neutral rotation and resting on a table.

Stabilization: Keeping force against the table with the mobilizing side forearm aids stabilization of the hand.

Mobilization: Grasp the distal segment of the joint to be manipulated with the index finger posteriorly and thumb anteriorly. For an anterior glide, apply a force toward the palm, creating an anterior glide. For a posterior glide, apply a force using the thumb toward the backside of the palm, creating a posterior glide.

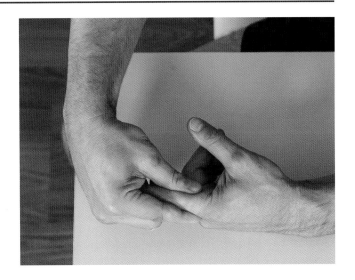

Goal of technique: To improve finger mobility. An anterior glide will help with flexion; a posterior glide will help with extension.

Notes: The closed packed position of the second through fifth MCP joints is full flexion. That of the PIP and DIP joints is full extension. Keeping the joint out of the closed packed position will allow more joint play. Additionally, oscillation of the distraction might decrease pain.

Lateral Glide for Hip Flexion in Kneeling

Client position: Standing, foot on stationary bench or chair.

Stabilization: Client grasps the bench or chair with bilateral hands.

Mobilization: A sheet or strap is placed around client's proximal thigh/groin region and attached to a stationary structure. A towel or weightlifting belt can be placed in this region and then attached to the sheet or strap for comfort. Client is asked to flex hip via moving trunk/upper body down toward floor (e.g., pelvic on femoral hip flexion) while maintaining the lateral distraction force of the sheet or strap.

Goal of technique: To increase pain-free hip flexion motion.

Note: This technique can be performed without the lateral distraction, although it may be required to abduct and externally rotate the hip farther to avoid pain.

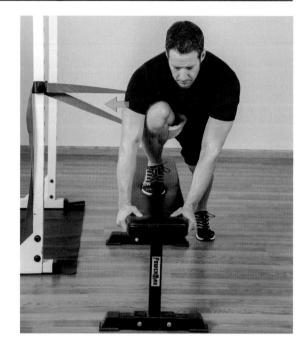

Lateral Glide for Hip Flexion in a Squat Position

Client position: Standing next to a stationary surface.

Stabilization: Client's body serves as stabilization.

Mobilization: A sheet or strap is placed around client's proximal thigh/groin region and attached to a stationary structure. A towel or weightlifting belt can be placed in this region and then attached to the sheet or strap for comfort. Client is asked to squat (e.g., pelvic on femoral hip flexion) as tolerated while maintaining the distraction force from the sheet or strap.

Goal of technique: To increase pain-free squatting motion.

Notes: The sheet or strap will need to be adjusted so it provides the necessary distraction in the location of client's pain (e.g., the strap will likely need to be close to parallel to the floor at the depth of client's squat where they have pain).

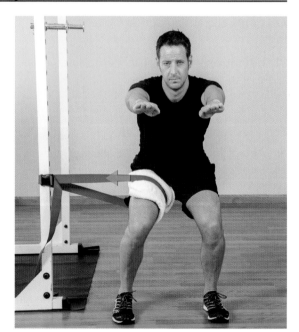

Hip Distraction in Quadruped

VIDEO A.2 **in the web study guide shows this technique.**

Client position: Kneeling on comfortable surface.

Stabilization: Client's body serves as stabilization.

Mobilization: A sheet or strap is placed around client's proximal thigh/groin region and attached to a stationary structure. A towel or weightlifting belt can be placed in this region and then attached to the sheet or strap for comfort. Client actively performs hip internal rotation as tolerated while maintaining the distraction force from the sheet or strap.

Goal of technique: To increase hip internal rotation with hip flexion.

Note: Increasing the amount of hip flexion and weight bearing on the involved side will likely limit the available hip internal rotation motion, but might be necessary for client.

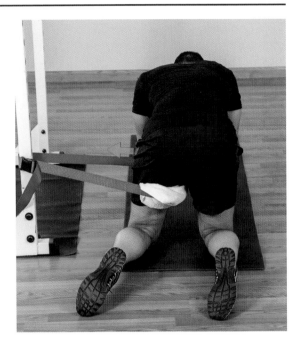

Hip Distraction in Standing With Hip Flexion

Client position: Standing with foot on a stable surface so hip is at approximately 90° flexion.

Stabilization: Client's body serves as stabilization.

Mobilization: A sheet or strap is placed around client's proximal thigh/groin region and attached to a solid, stationary structure. A towel or weightlifting belt can be placed in this region and then attached to the sheet or strap for comfort. Client actively pulls knee into hip adduction from this flexed position as tolerated while maintaining the distraction force from the sheet or strap.

Goals of technique: To increase limited hip adduction and internal rotation in hip flexion. A secondary goal is to reduce pain in this position.

Notes: By adducting the knee, the hip will internally rotate. Increasing hip flexion and weight bearing on the involved side will likely limit available hip internal rotation and adduction motion, but might be necessary for client.

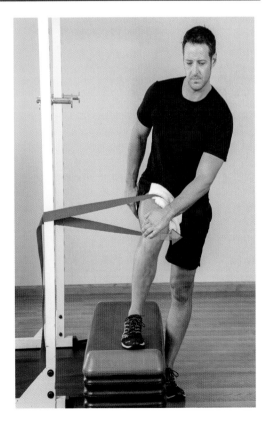

Long-Sitting Medial and Lateral Patellar Glides

Client position: Long-sitting with knee on a firm or padded surface, quadriceps relaxed.

Stabilization: The weight of client's leg serves as stabilization.

Mobilization: Client uses thumbs to passively glide the patella in a medial or lateral direction.

Goal of technique: To increase limited medial or lateral patellar gliding by stretching the superficial retinacular fibers.

Note: This mobilization is important following prolonged immobilization or after surgical procedures to the anterior knee.

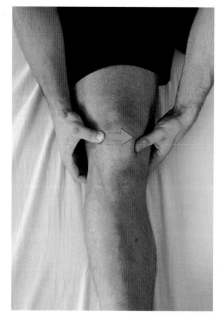
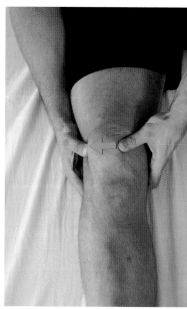

Long-Sitting Superior and Inferior Patellar Glides

Client position: Long-sitting with knee on a firm or padded surface, quadriceps relaxed.

Stabilization: The weight of client's leg serves as stabilization.

Mobilization: Client uses thumbs to passively glide the patella in a superior or inferior direction.

Goal of technique: To increase limited superior or inferior patellar gliding by stretching the superficial retinacular fibers, quadriceps tendon, and patellar tendon.

Note: This mobilization is important following prolonged immobilization or after surgical procedures to the anterior knee.

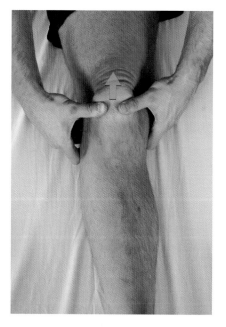
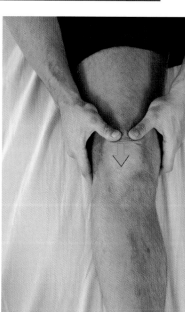

Medial and Lateral Patellar Tilt

Client position: Long-sitting with knee on a firm or padded surface, quadriceps relaxed.

Stabilization: The weight of client's leg serves as stabilization.

Mobilization: Client uses thumbs to passively tilt the patella medially or laterally.

Goal of technique: To increase limited lateral or medial tilting by stretching the deep retinacular fibers.

Notes: This mobilization is important following prolonged immobilization or after surgical procedures to the anterior knee. It might also be helpful following a lateral release procedure or in clients with excessive lateral pressure syndrome.

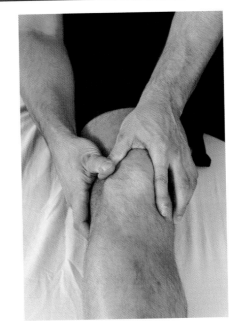
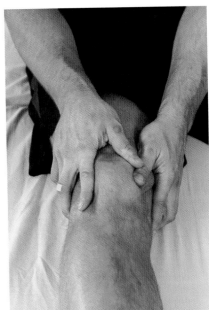

Weight-Bearing Rotation of the Tibia

Client position: Standing with affected leg's foot on stool or chair.

Stabilization: Client's weight through leg serves as stabilization.

Mobilization: Client uses hands grasped around tibia to passively rotate tibia, either internally while flexing knee or externally while extending knee.

Goal of technique: To directly assist client's functional movement through active knee flexion/extension.

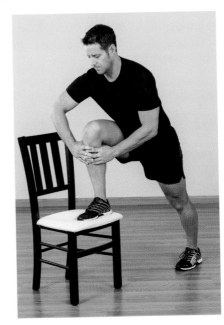
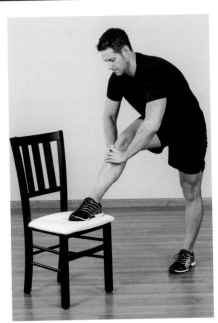

Talocrural Joint Distraction

Client position: Lying on back on floor, propped up on elbows.

Stabilization: Use a nonelastic strap wrapped in figure-8 fashion around ankle and attached to a stationary object.

Mobilization: Client moves away from the strapped ankle until a slight pull is felt in the ankle.

Goal of technique: To increase general motion at the ankle.

Note: A small towel under the strap can provide comfort from the strap pressure.

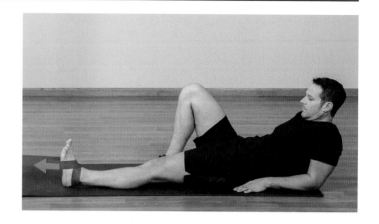

Posterior Talar Glide

 VIDEO A.3 in the web study guide shows this technique.

Client position: Standing with treated foot on a stable stool or chair depending on hip mobility (a stool is more appropriate for a relatively inflexible or painful hip).

Stabilization: A nonelastic strap is placed across the front of the ankle and secured to a stationary piece of furniture or floor beam.

Mobilization: The stool is situated so the slack of the strap is removed and a posterior pull is felt on the ankle.

Goal of technique: To increase ankle dorsiflexion.

Note: Moving into dorsiflexion will improve the effectiveness of the technique.

Lateral Calcaneal Glide

Client position: Seated with mobilizing leg crossed over opposite thigh.

Stabilization: The stabilizing hand grasps the front of the ankle joint.

Mobilization: The manipulating hand grips the posterior calcaneus, and palm of that hand applies a downward force that imparts a lateral glide to the calcaneus.

Goal of technique: To increase subtalar joint eversion.

Note: Ensure the client understands the glide is translatory, not rotational.

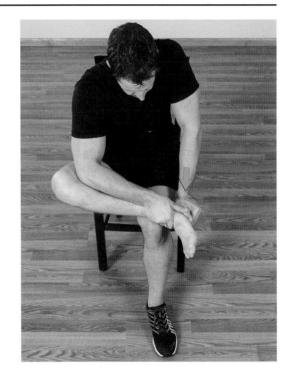

Great Toe Metatarsophalangeal (MTP) Distraction

Client position: Seated with mobilizing leg crossed over opposite thigh.

Stabilization: The stabilizing hand grasps the distal metatarsal using thumb on plantar surface and fingers on dorsal surface.

Mobilization: The manipulating hand grasps the proximal phalanx of the first toe. The mobilizing hand gently pulls the phalanx away from the fixed metatarsal, creating a distraction of the first MTP joint.

Goals of technique: This technique is used to improved general MTP mobility. Also, oscillation of the distraction might decrease pain.

Note: A manipulative thrust may be applied in a similar manner.

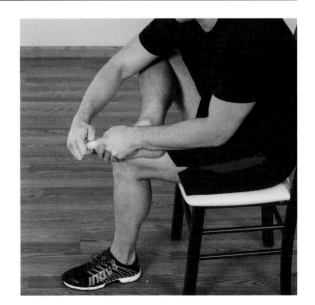

Clinical tip: A self-mobilization similar to that described for great toe MTP distraction can be applied to the other toes and the fingers at both the proximal and distal joints. Clients should ensure one hand is stabilizing the proximal segment while the other distracts the distal component directly away from the joint surface.

REFERENCES

Chapter 1

American Physical Therapy Association. *Guide to Physical Therapist Practice*. AISBN: 978-1-931369-85-5, DOI: 10.2522/ptguide3.0_978-1-931369-85-5

Baeyens JP, Van Roy P, De Schepper A, Declercq G, Clarijs JP. Glenohumeral joint kinematics related to minor anterior instability of the shoulder at the end of the late preparatory phase of throwing. *Clin Biomech*. 2001;16(9):752–757.

Barak T, Rosen ER, Sofer R. Basic concepts of orthopaedic manual therapy. In: Gould JA, ed. *Orthopaedic and Sports Physical Therapy*, 2nd ed. St. Louis, MO: Mosby; 1990.

Bialosky JE, Bishop MD, Bialosky JE, et al. Spinal manipulative therapy has an immediate effect on thermal pain sensitivity in people with low back pain: a randomized controlled trial. *Phys Ther*. 2009;89(12):1292–1303.

Bishop MD, Beneciuk JM, George, SZ. Immediate reduction in temporal sensory summation after thoracic spinal manipulation. *Spine* 2011;11(5):440–446.

Bolton PS The somatosensory system of the neck and its effect on the central nervous system. *J Manipulative Physiol Ther*. 1998;21:553–563.

Cannon JT, Prieto GJ, Lee A, et al. Evidence for opioid and non-opiod forms of stimulation produced analgesia in the rat. *Brain Res*. 1982;243:315–321.

Christian GH, Stanton GJ, Sissons D, et al. Immunoreactive ACTH, beta-endorphin, and cortisol levels in plasma following spinal manipulative therapy. *Spine* 1988;13:141–147.

Colloca CJ, Keller TS, Harrison DE, Moore RJ, Gunzburg R, Harrison DD. Spinal manipulation force and duration affect vertebral movement and neuromuscular responses. *Clin Biomech*. 2006;21:254–262.

Coppieters MW, Alshami AM. Longitudinal excursion and strain in the median nerve during novel nerve gliding exercises for carpal tunnel syndrome. *J Orthop Res* 2007;25:972–980.

Coppieters MW, Butler DS. Do "sliders" slide and "tensioners" tension? An analysis of neurodynamic techniques and considerations regarding their application. *Man Ther*. 2007;13(3):213–221.

Coranoda RA, Gay CW, Bialosky JE, et al. Changes in pain sensitivity following spinal manipulation: a systematic review and meta-analysis. *J Electromyogr Kinesiol*. 2012;22:752–767.

Cross V, Leach CM, Fawkes CA, Moore AP. Patients' expectations of osteopathic care: a qualitative study. *Health Expect*. 2015;18(5):1114–1126.

Frankel VH, Burstein AH, Brooks DB. Biomechanics of internal derangement of the knee. Pathomechanics as determined by analysis of the instant centers of motion. *J Bone Joint Surg Am*. 1971;53(5):945–962.

Gal J, Herzog W, Kawchuk G, Conway PJ, Zhang YT. Movements of vertebrae during manipulative thrusts to unembalmed human cadavers. *J Manip Physiol Ther*. 1997;20:30–40.

George SZ, Bishop MD, Bialosky, JE, et al. Immediate effects of spinal manipulation on thermal pain sensitivity: an experimental study. *BMC Musculoskelet Disord*. 2006;7:68.

Groen GJ, Baljet B, Drukker J. Nerve and nerve plexuses of the human vertebral column. *Am J Anat*. 1990;188:282–296.

Hosobuchi Y, Adams JE, Linchitz R. Pain relief by electrical stimulation of the central gray matter in human and its reversal by naloxone. *Science* 1977;197:183–186.

Hsieh CY, Vicenzino B, Yang CH, Hu MH, Yang C. Mulligan's mobilization with movement for the thumb: a single case report using magnetic resonance imaging to evaluate the positional fault hypothesis. *Man Ther*. 2002;7:44–49.

Johnson AJ, Godges JJ, Zimmerman GJ, Ounanian LL. The effect of anterior versus posterior glide joint mobilization on external rotation range of motion in patients with shoulder adhesive capsulitis. *J Orthop Sports Phys Ther*. 2007;37(3):88–99.

Lewitt K. *Manipulative Therapy in Rehabilitation of the Local Motor System*. Boston, MA: Butterworth; 1985.

MacConaill MA, Basmajian JV. *Muscles and Movements: A Basis for Human Kinesiology*, Baltimore, MD: Williams and Wilkins; 1969.

Maher C, Latimer, J. Pain or resistance: the therapists' dilemma. *Aust J Physiother*. 1993;38:257–260.

McClure PW, Flowers KR. Treatment of limited shoulder motion: a case study based on biomechanical considerations. *Phys Ther*. 1992;72(12):929–936.

McLain RF, Pickar JG. Mechanoreceptor endings in human thoracic and lumbar facet joints. *Spine* 1998;23:168–173.

Reynolds DV. Surgery in the rat during electrical analgesia induced by focal brain stimulations. *Science* 1969;164:444–445.

Riley SP, Bialosky, J, Cote MP, Swanson, BT, Tafuto V, Sizer PS, Brismée JM. Thoracic spinal manipulation for musculoskeletal shoulder pain: Can an instructional set change patient expectation and outcome? *Man Ther*. 2015;20(3):469–474.

Rushton A, Beeton K, Jordaan R, Langendoen J, Levesque L, Maffey L, Pool J. *International Federations of Orthopaedic Manipulative Physical Therapists (IFOMPT): Educational Standards in Orthopaedic Manipulative Therapy*. IFOMPT; 2016.

Sammarco GJ, Burstein AH, Frankel, VH. Biomechanics of the ankle: a kinematic study. *Orthop Clin North Am.* 1973;4(1):75–96.

Sanders GE, Reinnert O, Tepe R, et al. Chiropractic adjustment manipulation on subjects with acute low back pain: visual analog scores and plasma beta-endorphin levels. *J Manip Physiol Ther.* 1990;13:391–395.

Tullberg T, Blomberg S, Branth B, Johnsson R. Manipulation does not alter the position of the sacroiliac joint. A roentgen stereophotogrammetric analysis. *Spine* 1998;23:1124–1128.

Vernon HT, Dhami MSI, Howley TP, et al. Spinal manipulation and beta-endorphin: a controlled study of the effects of a spinal manipulation on plasma beta-endorphin levels in normal males. *J Manip Physio Ther.* 1986;9(2):115–123.

Williams NH, Hendry M, Lewis R, et al. Psychological response in spinal manipulation (PRISM): a systematic review of psychological outcomes in randomized controlled trails. *Complement Ther Med.* 2007;15(4):271–283.

Wooden MH. Mobilization of the upper extremity. In: Donatelli R, Wooden MJ, eds. *Orthopaedic Physical Therapy*, New York, NY: Churchill Livingston; 1989.

Wright A. Hypoalgesic post-manipulative therapy: a review of a potential neurophysiological mechanism. *Man Ther.* 1995;1:11–16.

Yezierski RP. Somatosensory input to the periaqueductal gray: a spinal relay to a descending control center. In: Depaulis A, Bandler R, eds. *The Midbrain Periaqueductal Gray Matter.* New York, NY: Plenum Press; 1991.

Chapter 2

Cyriax J. *Textbook of Orthopaedic Medicine, Volume 1: Diagnosis of Soft Tissue Lesions.* 6th ed. London, England: Bailliere Tindall; 1975:76–77.

Dutton M: *Orthopedic Examination, Evaluation and Intervention.* New York, NY: McGraw-Hill; 2004.

Ernst E. Adverse effects of spinal manipulation: a systematic review. *J R Soc Med.* 2007;100(7): 330–338.

Hayes KW, Petersen C, Falconer J. An examination of Cyriax's passive motion tests with patients having osteoarthritis of the knee. *Phys Ther.* 1994;74:697–708.

Maitland GD, Hengeveld E, Banks K., eds. *G. Maitland's peripheral manipulation.* 4th ed. Oxford, UK: Butterworth-Heinemann; 2005.

Pentelka L, Hebron C, Shapleski R, Goldshtein I. The effect of increasing sets (within one treatment session) and different set durations (between treatment sessions) of lumbar spine posteroanterior mobilisations on pressure pain thresholds. *Man Ther.* 2012;17(6):526–30.

Puentedura EJ, O'Grady WH. Safety of thrust joint manipulation in the thoracic spine: a systematic review. *J Man Manip Ther.* 2015;23(3):154–161.

Reiman MP. *Orthopedic clinical examination.* Champaign, IL: Human Kinetics; 2016.

Snodgrass SJ, Rivett DA, Robertson VJ. Manual forces applied during posterior-to-anterior spinal mobilization: a review of the evidence. *J Manipulative Physiol Ther.* 2006;29(4):316–329.

Stevinson J, Ernst E. Risks associated with spinal manipulation. *Am J Sports Med.* 2002;112(7): 566–571.

Chapter 3

Armijo-Olivo S, Pitance L, Singh V, Neto F, Thie N, Michelotti A. Effectiveness of manual therapy and therapeutic exercise for temporomandibular disorders: systematic review and meta-analysis. *Phys Ther.* 2016;96(1):9–25. doi:10.2522/ptj.20140548

Calixtre LB, Moriera RF, Franchini GH, Alburquerque-Sendin F, Oliveira, AB. 2015. Manual therapy for the management of pain and limited range of motion in subjects with signs and symptoms of temporomandibular disorder: a systematic review of randomised controlled trials. *J Oral Rehab.* 2015;42(11):847–861. doi:10.1111/joor.12321

Crane PL, Feinberg L, Morris J. A multimodal physical therapy approach to the management of a patient with temporomandibular dysfunction and head and neck lymphedema: a case report. *J Man Manip Ther.* 2015;23(1):37–42. doi:10.1179/2042618612Y.0000000021

Martins WR, Blasczyk JC, Aparecida Furlan de Oliveira M, et al. Efficacy of musculoskeletal manual approach in the treatment of temporomandibular joint disorder: a systematic review with meta-analysis. *Man Ther.* 2016;21:10–17. doi:10.1016/j.math.2015.06.009

Chapter 4

Blauvelt CT, F.R.T. *A Manual of Orthopaedic Terminology.* 5th ed. St Louis, MO: Mosby; 1994.

Blanpied PR, Gross AR, Elliott JM, et al. Neck Pain: Revision 2016. Clinical practice guidelines linked to the international classification of functioning, disability, and health from the orthopedic section of the American physical therapy association. *J Orthop Sports Phys Ther.* 2016;46:A1–A83.

Bogduk N, Mercer S. Biomechanics of the cervical spine. I: normal kinematics. *Clin Biomech.* 2000;15:633.

Dvorak J, Panjabi M. Functional anatomy of the alar ligaments. *Spine* 1987;12:183.

Koebke J, Brade H. Morphological and functional studies on the lateral joints of the first and second cervical vertebrae in man. *Anat Embryol (Berl).* 1982;164:265–275.

Mercer, SR, Bogduk N. The joints of the cervical vertebral column. *J Orthop Sports Phys Ther.* 2001;31:174–182.

Panjabi M, Crisco JJ, Vasavada A. Mechanical properties of the human cervical spine as shown by three-dimensional load-displacement curves. *Spine* 1982;26:2692–2700.

Panjabi M, Oda T, Crisco J, Dvorak J, Grob D. Posture affects motion coupling patterns of the upper cervical spine. *J Orthop Res.* 1993;11:525–536.

Penning L. Normal movements of the cervical spine. *Am J Roentgenol.* 1978;130:317–326.

Reiman MP. *Orthopedic Clinical Examination.* Champaign, IL: Human Kinetics; 2016.

White AA, Johnson RM, Panjabi MM, et al. Biomechanical analysis of clinical stability in the cervical spine. *Clin Ortho.* 1975;109:85–96.

Wong JJ, Shearer HM, Mior S, et al. Are manual therapies, passive physical modalities, or acupuncture effective for the management of patients with whiplash-associated disorders or neck pain and associated disorders? An update of the bone and joint decade task force on neck pain and its associated disorders by the optima collaboration. *Spine* 2016;16(12):1598–1630. doi:10.1016/j.spinee.2015.08.024

Chapter 5

Bautmans I, Van Arken J, Van Mackelenberg M, Mets T. Rehabilitation using manual mobilization for thoracic kyphosis in elderly postmenopausal patients with osteoporosis. *J Rehab Med.* 2010;42(2):129–135.

Martinez-Segura R, De-la-Llave-Rincón AI, Ortega-Santiago R, Cleland JA, Fernández-de-Las-Peñas C. Immediate changes in widespread pressure pain sensitivity, neck pain, and cervical range of motion after cervical or thoracic thrust manipulation in patients with bilateral chronic mechanical neck pain: a randomized clinical trial. *J Orthop Sports Phys Ther.* 2012;42(9):806–814.

Strunce JB, Walker MJ, Boyles RE, Young BA. The immediate effects of thoracic spine and rib manipulation on subjects with primary complaints of shoulder pain. *J Man Manip Ther.* 2009;17(4):230–236.

Walser R, Meserve BB, Boucher TR. The effectiveness of thoracic spine manipulation for the management of musculoskeletal conditions: a systematic review and meta-analysis of randomized clinical trials. *J Man Manip Ther.* 2009;17(4):237–246.

Chapter 6

Bronfort G, Haas M, Evans RL, Bouter LM. Efficacy of spinal manipulation and mobilization for low back pain and neck pain: a systematic review and best evidence synthesis. *Spine* 2004;4(3):335–356.

Kamali F, Shokri E. The effect of two manipulative therapy techniques and their outcome in patients with sacroiliac joint syndrome. *J Body Mov Ther.* 2012;16(1):29–35.

Leininger B, Bronfort G, Evans R, Reiter T. Spinal manipulation or mobilization for radiculopathy: a systematic review. *Phys Med Rehabil Clin N Am.* 2011;22(1):105–125.

Powers CM, Beneck GJ, Kulig K, Landel RF, Fredericson M. Effects of a single session of posterior-to-anterior spinal mobilization and press-up exercise on pain response and lumbar spine extension in people with nonspecific low back pain. *Phys Ther.* 2008;88(4):485–493.

Slaven EJ, Goode AP, Coronado RA, Poole C, Hegedus EJ. The relative effectiveness of segment specific level and nonspecific level spinal joint mobilization on pain and range of motion: results of a systematic review and meta-analysis. *J Man Manip Ther.* 2013;21(1):7–17.

Chapter 7

Camarinos J., Marinko L. Effectiveness of manual physical therapy for painful shoulder conditions: a systematic review. *J Man Manip Ther.* 2010;17(4):206–215.

Desjardins-Charbonneau A, Roy JB, Dionne CE, Fremont P, MacDermid JC, Desmeules F. The efficacy of manual therapy for rotator cuff tendinopathy: A systematic review and meta-analysis. *J Orthop Sports Med.* 2015;45(5):330–350.

Gebremariam L, Hay EM, van der Sande R, Rinkle WD, Koes BW, and Huisstede BMA. Subacromial impingement syndrome—effectiveness of physiotherapy and manual therapy. *Br J Sports Med.* 2014;48:1202–1208.

Noten S, Meeus M, Stassigns G, Glabbeek FV, Verborgt O, and Struyf F. Efficacy of different types of mobilization techniques in patients with primary adhesive capsulitis of the shoulder: a systematic review. *Arch Phys Med Rehab.* 2016;97:815–825.

Page MJ, Green S, Kramer S, et al. Manual therapy and exercise for adhesive capsulitis (frozen shoulder). *Cochrane Database of Systematic Rev.* 2014;8: doi:10.1002/14651858.CD011275

Chapter 8

Heisier R, O'Brien, VH, Schwartz DA. The use of joint mobilization to improve clinical outcomes in hand therapy: A review of the literature. *J Hand Ther.* (2013);26:297–311.

Lin F, Kohli N, Perlmutter S, Lim D, Nuber GW, Makhsous M. Muscle contribution to elbow joint valgus stability. *J Shoulder Elbow Surg.* 2017;16:795–802.

Park MC, Ahmad CS. Dynamic contributions of the flexor pronator mass to elbow valgus stability. *J Bone Joint Surg Am.* 2004;86:2268–2274.

Chapter 9

Coyle J, Robertson V. Comparison of two passive mobilizing techniques following Colles' fracture: A multielement design. *Man Ther.* 1998;3(1):34–41.

Randall T, Portney L, Harris B. Effects of joint mobilization on joint stiffness and active motion of the metacarpal-phalangeal joint. *J Orthop Sports Phys Ther.* 1992;16(1):30–36.

Tal-Akabi A, Rushton A. An investigation to compare the effectiveness of carpal bone mobilisation and neurodynamic mobilisation as methods of treatment for carpal tunnel syndrome. *Man Ther.* 2000;5(4):214–222.

Villafañe JH, Cleland J, Fernández-de-Las-Peñas C. The Effectiveness of a Manual Therapy and Exercise Protocol in Patients With Thumb Carpometacarpal Osteoarthritis: A Randomized Controlled Trial. *J Orthop Sports Phys Ther*. 2013;43(4):204–213.

Chapter 10

Bennell KL, Egerton T, Martin J, et al. Effect of physical therapy on pain and function in patients with hip osteoarthritis: a randomized clinical trial. *Jama* 2014;311(19):1987–1997. doi:10.1001/jama.2014.4591

Beumer L, Wong J, Warden SJ, Kemp JL, Foster P, Crossley KM. Effects of exercise and manual therapy on pain associated with hip osteoarthritis: a systematic review and meta-analysis. *Br J Sports Med*. 2016;50(8):458–463. doi:10.1136/bjsports-2015-095255

Diamond LE, Dobson FL, Bennell KL, Wrigley TV, Hodges PW, Hinman RS. Physical impairments and activity limitations in people with femoroacetabular impingement: a systematic review. *Br J Sports Med*. 2015;49(4):230–242. doi:10.1136/bjsports-2013-093340

Enseki K, Harris-Hayes M, White DM, et al. Nonarthritic hip joint pain. *J Orthop Sports Phys Ther*. 2014;44(6):A1–32. doi:10.2519/jospt.2014.0302

Hoeksma HL, Dekker J, Ronday HK, et al. Comparison of manual therapy and exercise therapy in osteoarthritis of the hip: a randomized clinical trial. *Arthritis Rheumatol*. 2004;51(5):722–729. doi:10.1002/art.20685

Pinto D, Robertson MC, Hansen P, Abbott JH. Economic evaluation within a factorial-design randomised controlled trial of exercise, manual therapy, or both interventions for osteoarthritis of the hip or knee: study protocol. *BMJ Open* 2011;1(1):e000136. doi:10.1136/bmjopen-2011-000136

Reiman MP, Matheson JW. Restricted hip mobility: clinical suggestions for self-mobilization and muscle re-education. *Int J Sports Phys Ther*. 2013;8(5):729–740.

Romeo A, Parazza S, Boschi M, Nava T, Vanti C. Manual therapy and therapeutic exercise in the treatment of osteoarthritis of the hip: a systematic review. *Reumatismo* 2013;65(2):63–74. doi:10.4081/reumatismo.2013.63

Sampath KK, Mani R, Miyamori T, Tumilty S. The effects of manual therapy or exercise therapy or both in people with hip osteoarthritis: A systematic review and meta-analysis. *Clin Rehabil*. 2015;30(12)1141–1155. doi:10.1177/0269215515622670

Wright AA, Hegedus EJ, Taylor JB, Dischiavi SL, Stubbs AJ. Non-operative management of femoroacetabular impingement: A prospective, randomized controlled clinical trial pilot study. *J Sci Med Sport*. 2016;19(9):716–721.

Chapter 11

Abbott FH, Robertson MC, Chapple C, et al. Manual therapy, exercise therapy, or both, in addition to usual care, for osteoarthritis of the hip or knee: a randomized controlled trial. 1: clinical effectiveness. *Osteoarthr Cartil*. 2013;21:525–534.

Deyle GD, Allison SC, Matelel RL, et al. Physical therapy treatment effectiveness for osteoarthritis of the knee: A randomized comparison of supervised clinical exercise and manual therapy procedures versus a home exercise program. *Phys Ther*. 2005;85:1301–1317.

Deyle GD, Gill NW, Allison SC, Hando BR, Rochino, DA. Knee OA: Which patients are unlikely to benefit from manual PT and exercise? *J Fam Pract*. 2012;61:E1–E8.

Hunt MA, Di Ciacca SR, Jones IC, Padfield B, Birmingham TB. Effect of anterior tibiofemoral glides on knee extension during gait in patients with decreased range of motion after anterior cruciate ligament reconstruction. *Physiother Can*. (2010);62:235–241.

Silvernail JL, Gill NW, Tehyen DS, Allison SC. Biomechanical measures of knee joint mobilization. *J Man Manip Ther*. (2011);19:162–171.

Chapter 12

Cruz-Diaz D, Lomas VR, Osuna-Perez MC, Hita-Contreras F, Marinez-Amat A. Effects of joint mobilization on chronic ankle instability: a randomized controlled trial. *Disabil Rehabil*. 2015;37(7):601–610.

Denegar CR, Hertel J, Fonseca J. The effect of lateral ankle sprain on dorsiflexion range of motion, posterior talar glide, and joint laxity. *J Orthop Sports Phys Ther*. 2002;32(4):166–173.

Hoch MC, McKeon, PO. The effectiveness of mobilization with movement at improving dorsiflexion after ankle sprain. *J Sport Rehabil*. 2010;19(2):226–232.

Irwin TA. Tendon injuries of the foot and ankle. In: Miller MD, SR Thompson, eds. *DeLee and Drez's Orthopaedic Sports Medicine*. 4th ed. Philadelphia, PA: Elsevier Saunders; 2014:1408–1427.

Landrum EL, Kelln CB, Parente WR, Ingersoll CD, Hertel J. Immediate effects of anterior-to-posterior talocrural joint mobilization after prolonged ankle mobilization: a preliminary study. *J Man Manip Ther*. 2008;16(2):100–105.

Loudon JK, Reiman MP, Sylvain J. The efficacy of manual joint mobilisation/manipulation in treatment of lateral ankle sprains: a systematic review. *Br J Sports Med*. 2014;48(5):365–370.

Vicenzino B, Branjerdporn M, Teys P, Jordan K. Initial changes in posterior talar glide and dorsiflexion of the ankle after mobilization with movement in individuals with recurrent ankle sprain. *J Orthop Sports Phys Ther*36 2006;(7):464–471.

Whitman JM, Cleland JA, Mintken PE. Predicting short term response to thrust and nonthrust manipulation and exercise in patients post inversion ankle sprain. *J Orthop Sports Phys Ther*. 209;39(3):188–200.

Chapter 13

Brantingham J, Guiry S, Kretzmann H, Globe G, Kite V. A pilot study of the efficacy of a conservative chiropractic protocol using graded mobilization, manipulation and ice in the treatment of symptomatic hallux abductovalgus bunions. *Clin Chiropr*. 2005;8:117–133.

Celik D, Kus G, Sirma SO. Joint mobilization and stretching exercise vs. steroid injection in the treatment of plantar fasciitis: A randomized controlled study. *Foot Ankle Int*. 2016;37(2):150–156.

Cleland JA, Abbott JH, Kidd MO, et al. Manual physical therapy and exercise versus electrophysical agents and exercise in the management of plantar heel pain. A multicentered randomized clinical trial. *J Orthop Sports Phys Ther*. 2009;39(8):573–585.

Govender N, Kretzmann H, Price J, Brantingham J, Globe G. A single-blinded randomized placebo-controlled clinical trial of manipulation and mobilization in the treatment of Morton's neuroma. *J Am Chiropr Assoc*. 207;44:9–18.

Jennings J, Davies G. Treatment of cuboid syndrome secondary to lateral ankle sprains: a case series. *J Orthop Sports Phys Ther*. 2005;35(7):409–415.

Petersen S, Brantingham J, Kretzmann H. The efficacy of chiropractic adjustment in the treatment of primary metatarsalgia. *Eur J Chiropr*. 2003;49:267–279.

Shamus J, Shamus E, Gugel RN, Brucker BS, Skaruppa C. The effect of sesamoid mobilization, flexor hallucis strengthening, and gait training on reducing pain and restoring function in individuals with hallux limitus: a clinical trial. *J Orthop Sports Phys Ther*. 2004;34(7):368–376.

Shasua A, Flechter S, Avidan L, Ofir D, Melayev A, Kalichman L. The effect of additional ankle and midfoot mobilizations on plantar fasciitis: a randomized controlled trial. *J Orthop Sports Phys Ther*. 2015;45(4):265–272.

INDEX

Note: The italicized *f* and *t* following page numbers refer to figures and tables, respectively.

Robert C. Manske PT, DPT, MPT, MEd, SCS, ATC, CSCS, is a professor in the doctoral physical therapy program at Wichita State University (WSU) in Wichita, Kansas. He graduated from WSU with a bachelor of arts degree in physical education in 1991, received a master

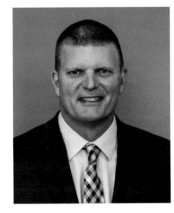

Courtesy of Jennifer E. Celso

of physical therapy degree in 1994, and earned a master of education degree in physical education in 2000. He received his DPT from Massachusetts General Institute of Health Professions in 2006.

Manske has been an APTA Board Certified Sports Physical Therapist since 2002, is a Certified Strength and Conditioning Specialist (CSCS) through the National Strength and Conditioning Association, and is a certified athletic trainer (ATC) through the Board of Certification for the Athletic Trainer. He was a two-term vice president of the APTA Sports Physical Therapy Section. He has received numerous awards for excellence in teaching at the local, state, and national levels, including the APTA Sports Physical Therapy Section's Excellence in Education Award in 2007 and the Ron Peyton Award in 2018.

Manske has published multiple books, chapters, articles, and home study courses related to orthopedic and sports rehabilitation, and he has been editor of nine books on various topics related to orthopedics and sports. He is an associate editor for *International Journal of Sports Physical Therapy* and is currently a manuscript reviewer for *Journal of Orthopedic and Sports Physical Therapy, Sports Health, Athletic Training and Sports Health Care, Physical Therapy in Sports,* and *American Journal of Sports Medicine (AJSM)*. From 2005 through 2007 and 2011 through 2017, he was a principle reviewer for *AJSM*.

Manske has lectured at the state and national levels during meetings for APTA, NATA, and NSCA. In addition to his full-time faculty appointment, he is a physical therapist and athletic trainer at Via Christi Health and also serves as a teaching associate for the University of Kansas Medical Center Department of Rehabilitation Sciences and for the Via Christi Family Practice Sports Medicine Residency Program.

B.J. Lehecka, DPT, is an assistant professor in the department of physical therapy in the College of Health Professions at Wichita State University (WSU) in Wichita, Kansas. At WSU, Lehecka teaches course work concerning the hip and spine regions, pos-

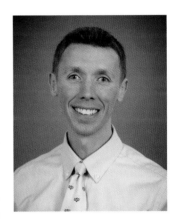

B.J. Lehecka

ture, gait, proprioceptive neuromuscular facilitation, musculoskeletal evaluation, and the treatment of musculoskeletal pathology. In 2016, he was awarded WSU's Rodenberg Award for Excellence in Teaching due to his outstanding work in the classroom.

Lehecka has published multiple peer-reviewed journal articles, authored and edited numerous book chapters, and presented at state, national, and international conferences. He earned his bachelor's degree in kinesiology from Kansas State University in 2006 and a doctorate in physical therapy from Wichita State University in 2009. Lehecka serves his community as a physical therapist and is a PhD candidate at Rocky Mountain University of Health Professions.

Michael P. Reiman, PT, DPT, MEd, OCS, SCS, ATC, FAAOMPT, CSCS, is an associate professor in the department of community and family practice at Duke University Medical Center in Durham, North Carolina. He is also part of the clinical faculty in the Duke

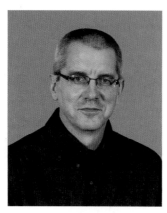

© Human Kinetics

University Medical Center manual therapy fellowship program. Reiman has published more than 50 articles in peer-reviewed journals as well as 10 book chapters and three home study courses. He coauthored *Functional Testing in Human Performance* (Human Kinetics, 2009) with Robert C. Manske. He has given numerous presentations at national, regional, and local conferences.

Reiman is a member of the American Physical Therapy Association, American Academy of Orthopaedic Manual Physical Therapists, Kansas Physical Therapy Association, National Athletic Trainers' Association, National Strength and Conditioning Association, and Alpha Eta Society. He serves as an associate editor for *Journal of Physical Therapy* and is a member of the editorial boards for *International Journal of Sports Physical Therapy* and *Journal of Sport Rehabilitation*. He is a reviewer for *British Journal of Sports Medicine*, *Journal of Sports Science and Medicine*, *Physiotherapy Theory and Practice*, *Journal of Sport Rehabilitation*, *Journal of Manual and Manipulative Therapy*, *Journal of Orthopaedic and Sports Physical Therapy*, *Clinical Anatomy*, and *Journal of Athletic Training*.

Reiman is a level 1 track and field coach and a level 1 Olympic weightlifting club coach. He also works as a strength and conditioning specialist for women's volleyball at Friends University in Wichita, Kansas, and for the men's and women's volleyball teams at Newman University in Wichita.

Reiman resides in Hillsborough, North Carolina, where he enjoys spending time with his family, hiking in the surrounding hills, and wakeboarding with his children.

Janice K. Loudon, PT, PhD, SCS, ATC, CSCS, is a professor in the department of physical therapy education at Rockhurst University in Kansas City, Missouri. She has more than 30 years of experience in clinical sports medicine and has worked as a physical therapy

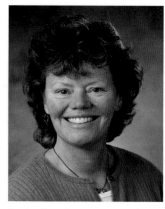

Janice Loudon

instructor for over 20 years. Dr. Loudon was previously an associate professor at Duke University and at the University of Kansas Medical Center in Kansas City.

Dr. Loudon is a board-certified sport physical therapist, certified athletic trainer, and certified strength and conditioning specialist. She is also a member of the National Athletic Trainers' Association (NATA) and the American Physical Therapy Association (APTA). She serves as the associate editor of the home study courses for APTA's Sports Physical Therapy Section.

Loudon has published multiple articles in peer-reviewed journals, written several book chapters, and coauthored *Clinical Mechanics and Kinesiology* (Human Kinetics, 2013) and two editions of *The Clinical Orthopedic Assessment Guide* (Human Kinetics, 1998, 2008). She is a frequent presenter at national, state, and local conferences.

Loudon resides in Overland Park, Kansas. In her spare time, she enjoys hiking, cycling, gardening, and rooting for the Kansas Jayhawks.